# THE WEIGHT OF THE WHITE COAT

# THE WEIGHT OF THE WHITE COAT

Latinos Navigating American Medicine

GLENDA M. FLORES

UNIVERSITY OF CALIFORNIA PRESS

University of California Press
Oakland, California

© 2025 by Glenda M. Flores

Cataloging-in-Publication data is on file at the Library of Congress.

ISBN 978-0-520-40921-7 (clot)
ISBN 978-0-520-40922-4 (pbk.)
ISBN 978-0-520-40924-8 (ebook)

GPSR Authorized Representative: Easy Access System Europe, Mustamäe tee 50, 10621 Tallinn, Estonia, gpsr.requests@easproject.com

34   33   32   31   30   29   28   27   26   25
10   9   8   7   6   5   4   3   2   1

*Para mis padres, Rome y Ricardo.*
*This book is dedicated to the families that lost a loved one to the*
*COVID-19 pandemic.*

# Contents

# List of Tables and Figures

# Acknowledgments

WHEN I WROTE a Vivencias Report, a short personal essay focused on STEM curriculum in public schools, for the interdisciplinary journal *Latino Studies* titled "Latino/as in the Hard Sciences: Increasing Latina/o Participation in Science, Technology, Engineering, and Math (STEM) Related Fields" over a decade ago, I did not think that those initial ruminations would turn into a full-fledged book. That piece was originally inspired by my Mexican immigrant father's career aspirations for me. I thought my father wanted me to become an elementary school teacher, but he told me he wanted me to reach for the stars and become an astronaut. He would have liked to become a surgeon had he been able to attend college. The idea of studying Latinas/os in STEM careers was alluring to me, and when I found that several of the women I interviewed for my first book on Latina teachers had degrees in computer science, mathematics, and biology, I knew I had a new seven-year project to work on.

This research on Latina/o physicians could not have been completed without the unwavering support of faculty in the Department of Chicano/Latino Studies at UC Irvine, whose expertise on the social determinants of health in communities of color is unmatched. The conversations that I've had with Drs. Belinda Campos, Alana LeBrón, and Isabel F. Almeida enhanced the book's analysis.

Research trips to Cuba, Mexico, and Puerto Rico add texture to the story. A research trip with UC-Cuba, an organization helmed by Professors Anita Casavantes-Bradford and Raul Fernández, exposed me to Cuba's medical diplomacy program. I came across more women scientists than ever. I met women who were architects, biochemists, doctors, and engineers. This first trip inspired me to take a medical Spanish and sociocultural understandings of medicine course at the Instituto Cultural Oaxaca in Oaxaca, Mexico. I loved learning about *parteras* [midwives] from my Zapotec teacher Zuly Reyes, who fused both Indigenous and institutionalized forms of medicine in our course. Dr. Victor M. Rodriguez gave me a brief overview of physicians practicing in Puerto Rico. A visiting scholar position at the University of Hawai'i at Mānoa in the Gender and Sexuality Studies Department greatly helped me develop my thoughts on gender and colorism. Professors Monisha DasGupta and Vernadette Gonzalez provided invaluable support.

Sociologists Pierrette Hondagneu-Sotelo, Lata Murti, Gilda Ochoa, Irene Browne, Jody Agius Vallejo, Adia Harvey Wingfield, and Jazmín Muro read drafts and gave me insightful feedback. I also benefited greatly from the support from colleagues across disciplinary fields such as Drs. Adriana Briscoe, Nancy Burke, Long Bui, Chuck Vega, and John Billimeck. Nancy Fernández, Catherine Osborne, Kate Epstein, and Naomi Schneider also read pieces and helped me strengthen my claims.

My women of color writing group that included stellar sociologists Drs. Amada Armenta, Rocío Rosales, Irene Vega, Sylvia Zamora, and Mirian Martínez-Aranda read multiple drafts and greatly improved the overall contribution of this book. All of us have benefited from the Creative Connections: Writing and Meditation Retreat that helped us adopt a healthy lifestyle by providing us with nutritious meals and time in nature as we crafted our projects. At this retreat, I met Drs. Shanondora Billiot, Rosalba Resendez, Kate Wegman, Natasha Howard, Eileen Díaz McConnell, and Nadia Kim, who all provided a wealth of laughs and critical feedback. Drs. Tanya Golash Boza and Ayu L. Saraswati created this space for us to thrive and I have to thank them both as well as Dr. Sabrina Strings for commissioning pieces from me that pushed the theoretical contributions of my work. These opportunities were made possible because of the networks the retreat cultivates.

Yoselinda Mendoza and Thalía Fabian began this research with me when they were both stellar undergraduates, and the project was just an idea. The former received her PhD in sociology from Cornell University, and the latter is currently completing medical school to become a doctor. Both exceeded my expectations, and I know they will accomplish tremendous feats in the world. I used this project to mentor and train other undergraduate students who wanted to learn the art of coding and writing analytical memos: Jaileen Gutierrez, Teresa Ramírez, Joceline Porron, Lesley Marizol Noguez, Daniela Fox, and Andrea Serrano provided me with helpful research assistance. As the project progressed, Maricela Bañuelos, a doctoral student in sociology, helped me organize all of my data onto new online coding platforms. She is a whiz at it!

This research could not have been completed without generous support from several internal and external funding agencies. Early support for this research project came from the UC/All Campus Consortium on Research for Diversity (UC/ACCORD), which helped me to begin interviewing women physicians. This research also received financial support from the prestigious Hellman Foundation, which allowed me to expand my study and include men. At UCI, I am immensely grateful that I received a SPIRIT grant from the Office of

Inclusive Excellence, support from the Interim Covid-19 Research Recovery Program, and the Associate Professor Research Award from the School of Social Sciences made possible by the Dean's Leadership Society. I also owe a big thank you to Miguel Macias, the Mexican-American artist who crafted the cover image for the book. The prayer candle has many meanings—such as lighting someone's way or praying for a loved one's health and speedy recovery. I send a virtual hug to Lucero Zamudio, the UCI School of Medicine's Program Coordinator for the Program in Medical Education for the Latino Community (PRIME-LC), for including me in the educational trips that medical students take over the summer.

My brother Ricky Flores works as a dentist for a migrant community in northern California, and he connected me to several physicians he knew. Ricky also came to my PRIME-LC MS1 class and discussed the importance of oral health. Thanks, Rick! My mother was a key informant when she connected me to physicians during her medical appointments. Jorge, known as "Gorgie Pie," provided endless laughs and encouraged me to use more adjectives in my prose. "Yes, Gorgie. I'm done with my book now." Thank you, "G."

Lastly, I also want to thank the Latina/o physicians who donated their time to this project, without whom this research would not be possible. The COVID-19 pandemic hit as I was in the midst of data collection. Many of the doctors included here were on the front lines, working in the most afflicted communities that were disproportionately their own. At the heart of this book are several of them, who were there before, and remain in the occupation today.

# 1.

# THE WHITE COAT'S POLYVALENCE

ROSA DURAN BECAME a part of her Mexican immigrant father's health care team at age seven. She recounted that experience many years later when we talked about her medical career: "My world turned upside down when he suffered brain damage." Now a family medicine practitioner, Rosa recalled that as a child she regularly "tagged along" with her mother to her father's medical appointments. Her mother did not want to leave her in the care of her four older brothers, the oldest of whom was only fourteen at the time. She also could not afford a nanny. Eventually, Rosa became a vital part of her ailing father's care, often completing tasks that neither parent could perform. Rosa was the primary interlocutor[1] between the family and the medical establishment. As a language broker—a term used to describe the children of immigrants who are skilled in two vernaculars–she translated complex medical jargon from doctors and nurses during office visits and hospitalizations. She also managed her father's medication dosages at home. Through tears running down her rosy cheeks, she told me about the toll her father's disability, illness, and eventual death years later took on the family. So heavy was this emotional weight that two minutes into our conversation, I sat across from a sobbing Latina doctor in her place of work. When I looked down at my interview questions, I realized I had only asked the first one.

Despite these early hardships, Dr. Rosa Duran felt that she reaped the benefits of being the youngest in the family. Her mother, an "ironing queen" at work—as Rosa referred to her due to the speed with which she pressed clothes—paid for her to attend a private Catholic high school in Northridge, California. Her father's illness informed many of her higher education decisions, such as commuting from Northridge to UCLA, the institution where she earned her baccalaureate degree in Physiological Science and then her medical degree. Her medical brokering served as a valuable socio-cultural skill en route to medical school. At thirty-six years old, she now worked at a large teaching hospital near downtown Los Angeles. Rosa reflected, "There is a special little pocket for us [bilingual and college-educated Latinas] because there's not enough of us in such a huge population." Latina physicians are only 2.4 percent of all doctors in the United States and most of them are younger and bilingual women.[2] Like Rosa, they are carving out a space in a profession that has traditionally been the domain of white men in America.

Demographic trends in the medical profession show that a small but growing number of Latinas/os[3] are making inroads into science, technology, engineering, and mathematics (STEM) career fields such as medicine. Latino men make up 3.6 percent of all doctors in the United States.[4] Dr. Lorenzo Servando Contreras is one of them. In contrast to the public hospital Dr. Duran worked in, he worked at a private practice in an upscale coastal community of Los Angeles. His specialty was surgery. In our interview, Lorenzo pondered the dual lives he lived over the course of his career. At over six feet—and a former Marine—he towered over my five-foot-two frame. Lorenzo told me that he "was enlisted" into the military upon high school graduation, not so much by choice. Military recruiters were a common sight in the high school he attended in La Puente, California, a community east of downtown Los Angeles that is over 80 percent Latine. He did not want to take the vocational route that was presented to him by school counselors, and the GI Bill's financial incentives swayed him. As the oldest child, he felt an obligation to provide financially for his parents, who worked in low-wage jobs. The Marines gave him extensive training in STEM areas, especially technology, computer science, and first aid, subjects he was not exposed to in high school.

The military also exposed Lorenzo to blatant forms of racism that he had to defend himself from physically. In the Marines, he told me, "was the only time I have ever been called a spick, ever been called a wetback, the only time I had to fight [racist] people . . . punch people [because of the racism]." Now he sat in an upscale office in what appeared to be a very profitable practice. The explicit and confrontational racism he experienced then was a far cry from the more subtle forms he experienced as a reconstructive surgeon. His hiring, however, had been problematic. Lorenzo was hired as an independent contractor by the owner of the practice because he could attract a "diverse clientele." Yet one of his colleagues, a white male surgeon, did not want Lorenzo to advertise his middle name in the practice signage because it was "too Mexican" sounding. Lorenzo resisted and hung up his diplomas, a Bachelor of Science in Physiology and a medical degree, both from UCLA and that proudly displayed his entire name, in his office.

Rosa and Lorenzo's stories were fascinating to me, and after many interviews I saw how the complex and cumulative weights of gender and ethnicity played a significant and patterned role across their familial, educational, and workplace trajectories. Like feminist and intersectionalities scholars[5] before me, in this book, I take an intersectional and curious feminist lens to examine how gender-based discrimination produces markedly different experiences for men and women physicians who self-identify in the Latina/o pan-ethnic category and work in a predominantly white and masculinized high-skill occupation. An intersectional lens reveals how the interlinked nature of various social locations—such as gender, race, class, generational status, legal status, and country of medical school training,[6]—produce a vast array of outcomes that shift over time and place across organizations for bicultural people.[7] I show how this process unfolds for individuals who fall under the all-encompassing label of Latinidad.[8]

To be sure, Rosa and Lorenzo share many similarities. Both are the US-born children of working-class Mexican immigrants; they are the first in their families to attend and graduate from college, self-described as Spanish/English bilingual, attended a top-tier public university, majored in the same field, and went to the same US medical school at different points in time. However, Rosa ultimately entered a feminized specialty and Lorenzo a more masculinized one in ways that mirror larger gendered specialty selection patterns. After all, women make up a larger percentage of residents in family medicine and pediatrics while men prefer to specialize in surgery and radiology.[9] More generally, both Latinas and Latinos have higher representation in primary care than other specialties.[10] Primary care physicians in a given area have been linked to improved population mortality as they serve as stewards of care.[11]

Rosa and Lorenzo's school-to-work transitions were a point of contrast. Rosa realized that her bilingualism was a valuable cultural asset and linguistic skill that was rewarded, granting her medical training opportunities in ways that were not readily available for Lorenzo.[12] Being a language broker formed an important foundation for her linguistic capital. Bilingualism is positively associated with high school completion and occupational prestige among Latinas, but oral and passive bilingualism—childhood exposure to a language but little command of it—are negatively associated with high school completion among men.[13] Men who speak Spanish may be stigmatized in public spaces, whereas bilingual women may gain valuable skills that are rewarded in school and the labor market. Rosa and Lorenzo's patient base was also a point of contrast. Rosa had a mostly Spanish-speaking and marginalized patient base; Lorenzo's patients were mostly English-dominant and affluent. She worked for a large health maintenance organization (HMO) that gave her benefits and a schedule that she felt allowed her to better balance being a professional working mother than other options. Lorenzo, on the other hand, was looking into creating an S corporation—a small business—to establish his private practice in partnership with a fellow Latino surgeon who specialized in trauma.

How does gender inform the pathways that various Latina/o heritage doctors take into US medicine and how does it influence their professional work lives? *The Weight of the White Coat* finds answers to this question by looking within the contours of Latinidad to shed light on the cumulative weight of intersecting identities such as gender, class, and phenotype within the same pan-ethnic group, all of which coalesce to make the job more challenging for some as they go through it—limiting their advancement—and propelling others forward. I use a qualitative approach to examine within-group patterns in light of larger US inequities among the participants who fall within a single pan-ethnic category in large national data sets. Data sets such as the American Medical Association Physician Masterfile do not include measures of race-ethnicity, and these are crucial to understanding intra-Latina/o dynamics and intricacies among doctors. I argue that linguistic capital is one such intricacy, heavily tied to opportunity structures, that help us weigh the equity tasks inconspicuously assigned to them. I contend that for Latina/o doctors the weight of the white coat is polyvalent, and produces varied configurations of oppression, opportunity, and privilege as they make their career choices and move across familial, educational, and medical institutions in America. This weight also communicates gravity, respect, and responsibility, commanding respect from co-ethnic patients and their families, who recognize it, when bilingual Latina/o doctors wear it, as an antidote to the medical racism that Latines face.

## WHAT WE KNOW ABOUT THE MEDICAL PROFESSION AND LATINES IN HEALTH

In their book *Boys in White* (1976), qualitative ethnographers Howard Becker, Blanche Geer, Everett C. Hughes, and Anselm L. Strauss argued that the significant pressures of medical school training outweighed prior roles and experiences. Their groundbreaking book revealed that socio-demographic characteristics such as class background had little or no impact on program completion in the face of the overwhelming medical student culture and requirements.[14] At the same time, the "boys in white" held deficient perspectives of women and poor patients. Medical school pedagogy and culture reproduced white heteropatriarchy, the notion that heterosexuality and patriarchy are the norm for doctors and the people they try to heal. Their study focused on white and monolingual English-speaking men in the rural Midwest in Kansas, whereas I focus on fully licensed Latina/o doctors who work with diverse marginalized and affluent communities in rural and urban locales all over California.

A holistic account of the lives of Latina/o physicians would not be complete without bringing in the historical sociopolitical context that affects the co-ethnic patients with whom they interact day after day. As I conducted the interviews, it was common to hear of physicians serving as interpreters for their parents, especially women. Interpreters serve in part as a shield against poor care. To be sure, Latine immigrants to the United States have frequently experienced degrading, even violent care in a system designed for English speakers not deemed racial others, and several high-profile cases make it difficult for them to establish trust in US-based doctors. In the early 1900s, US public health officials marked Mexicans as having poor hygiene and as carriers of contagion.[15] Government-sponsored hygienic interventions in Los Angeles supposedly designed to promote assimilation to US culture reflected the patronizing and humiliating, if nominally beneficent, treatment of Mexican immigrants in that period. When public opinion shifted during the Great Depression in the 1930s, Mexicans were scapegoated for the country's economic ills and seen as carriers of disease and thus deportable, whether or not they had persisting ties to Mexico. In the 1940s American agricultural growers' demand for Mexican men for farm work led to the Bracero Program (1942–1964), under which laborers seeking economic prosperity were dehumanized during physical examinations. As historian Natalia Molina writes, applicants for the program "were asked to strip and then were sprayed with a white powder on their hair, face, and [most humiliatingly their] 'lower area.'"[16] Gasoline and DDT pesticides were used during these examinations without gathering informed consent.

Throughout history, medical professionals have also been active participants in controlling fertility rates and childrearing practices of Latinas.[17] The US government sponsored the widespread sterilization of women and girls on the island of Puerto Rico during the 1950s and '60s, and Spanish-speaking immigrant Latinas faced forced sterilization in Los Angeles medical facilities during the 1970s.[18] In Puerto Rico coercion was largely economic; in Los Angeles it included misinformation, putting consent forms for tubal ligations before women while they were in labor or heavily sedated, and denying them medical care until they signed. When patients fought back, suing for damages in 1978 based on the violation of their rights, the state court ruled largely in the hospital's favor. This was despite a cultural anthropologist's testimony that the doctors of the Women's Hospital at Los Angeles County+USC Medical Center, under the leadership of Dr. James Quilligan, had used eugenics-based arguments to justify their actions. The state court accepted the defense's argument that doctors could not be expected to obtain sufficient cultural competence quickly enough to avoid forced sterilization. The only positive outcome of the case was that the court ruled that consent forms had to be given in a language that a patient could understand. Cases like this one illustrate the practices of the boys in white in medicine. We know much less about the journeys that Latinas/os undertake before donning the white coat. And once they receive it, how they carry the weight of that coat.

## THE WEIGHT OF THE WHITE COAT

*La bata blanca*, the white coat, is the doctor's signature garment.[19] To signal a transition from "quackery" and medieval medicine in the 1800s, physicians began to don a white coat, a symbol of cleanliness and purity that showed respect for science. At contemporary medical schools across the nation budding doctors participate in the white-coat ceremony, in which they are presented with their coats and recite the Hippocratic Oath in unison.[20] This is the moment where they signal their commitment to provide compassionate care to patients "objectively" and without bias. For Latina/o doctors, to greater and lesser degrees, the white coat has a polyvalent weight. This weight is not measured in grams or ounces. Rather, I argue that the intersections of various social locations fall on a spectrum that fluctuates for Latina/o doctors and shifts over time, place, and across institutions as they move up the medical hierarchy. These multivalent weights are context-contingent and reflect larger patterns of advantage and disadvantage that may not be visible to all members of society but are certainly observed, felt, and reproduced. In some contexts, they are oppressive, heavy, and burdensome. In other phases of life and across institutions, the inverse may happen, where the intersection of particular social categories that STEM fields and medicine already privilege garner influence, respect, rewards, and resource allocation. Latina/o physicians are not a monolith, and the white coat's multivalence is not dispersed equally among them. Indeed, sometimes participants themselves brushed off their marginalization because of the high social status accorded to physicians and the salary they earn. Gender inequality curiously shifts as bilingual Latina/o doctors transition from beginning medical students to fully licensed practitioners.[21]

All of these registers occur within the context of efforts to diversify medicine in a changing and corporatized medical landscape. All of them work in a racial capitalist system that extracts resources from different people.[22] In the case of Latina/o doctors in a corporatized medical industry, this resource is often their linguistic capital. Linguistic capital is valuable. However, a racial capitalist system makes it difficult to advocate for one another when certain tasks are systematically assigned to particular groups, subtly maintaining and reproducing status hierarchies. Assessing the effects of a profit-driven industry on doctors is not the main focus of my book, but Latina/o physicians are entering the profession at a time of major changes. In "rank" doctors are changing from self-employed to being employed by large organizations.[23] There is also an influx of international medical physicians of color and increasing diversification efforts. Despite these organizational changes, Latina/o doctors face an organizational inertia due to larger structural constraints and status biases enforced by various social actors that continue to uphold white masculinist standards that have dominated STEM education and institutions for centuries.

Occupational sex segregation remains a defining feature of the US medical profession. "Physicianhood" in the US is conceived of as masculine due to the sheer gender imbalance in the profession even though women have made steady gains.[24] White men are at the top of the doctor hierarchy in American medicine, and, at 44.4 percent of the profession they still represent a plurality.[25] Women make up 36.1 percent of the active doctor workforce overall, and white women are 21.4 percent of physicians.[26] When medical student and journalist Anna Goshua wrote about the weight of the white coat for the *Journal of the American Medical Association*, she detailed the jitters she felt during her first standardized patient encounter as a novice woman medical student in training. She described contorting and molding her behaviors into what she believed "a doctor-to-be should be like" in ways similar to the white women doctors in Judith Lorber's *Women Physicians: Careers, Status and Power*.[27] Lorber, writing in the early 1980s, noted that continuous and informal small acts of devaluation and familial obligations prevented white women doctors from reaching the top echelons of the professional hierarchy in the 1980s. White men doctors had a clear gender advantage over them, especially when it came to demonstrations of respect and deference.

Joan Cassell's 1998 *The Woman in the Surgeon's Body*, too, described how an unequal gender hierarchy was produced in surgical specialties that privilege a more masculine culture. This masculinized culture placed women surgeons in a subordinate status in the Midwest and East Coast. Cassell showed that women nurses were deferential to male surgeons, for example by helping them with gowns and gloves before operations, a service the nurses denied to white women surgeons. Nurses also frequently questioned white women surgeons about their expertise. In short, nurses, often acted as "enforcers of gender-appropriate behavior" and white women surgeons continued to face sexism in the profession.[28] These studies of white men and women were presented as universal and applicable to everyone regardless of race, ethnicity, or specialty.

While I am not the first scholar to use the white coat as a symbol of "physicianhood," I am the first to provide a gendered account of its uneven and cumulative weight on mostly multilingual Latina/o physicians and how that weight varies across their journey from parental messages about the career and into practice. The people you will meet in this book are from heterogeneous backgrounds and mostly work in communities that serve predominantly poor immigrant and racial/ ethnic minority families in various hospitals, clinics, and medical offices all over California—the state that employs the largest share of active physicians. A smaller number of them work as plastic surgeons or medical concierges in places like Beverly Hills[29] and serve affluent and wealthy patients and communities.

I wrote this book in part to probe what makes it possible (and probable) for Latina/o physicians to enter and remain in the profession. The metaphor of the leaky pipeline has been used to describe some of the barriers: underrepresented groups pursuing degrees in STEM-related fields trailing off and exiting at important junctures before reaching the end goal of majoring in these fields, such as earning a biology degree, applying to medical school, obtaining a medical degree, and performing the duties of a doctor in a medical facility. Addressing the leaks involves looking at what it takes to persist, how someone starts to fall through the leaks in the pipeline but gets back on course, and what occurs on the job, post-degree.

## WHY LATINA/O PHYSICIANS?

The American Medical Association (AMA), established in 1847, is the premier organization for all doctors; yet, it has an opprobrious history of explicitly excluding women and Black doctors,[30] and doctors of Latina/o heritage have noticeably been missing from the conversation. The National Hispanic Medical Association (NHMA, established in 1994), an ethnic network and important source of information for Latina/o heritage physicians, emerged almost a hundred and fifty years after the AMA. The composition of the organization was referenced by Dr. Olga Rivera, in internal medicine and an active member of the NHMA: "It's a very different situation for the Latina/o doctors that I know that are part of our [medical] organization . . . [W]e're all the first-time families that go to college." At almost 20 percent of the US

TABLE I

Top Five States of Active Physicians Who Identify as Hispanic, Latino, or of Spanish Origin (Alone or in Combination), 2020

| Rank | State | Number | Percentage |
|------|-------|--------|------------|
| 1 | Florida | 9,309 | 18% |
| 2 | Texas | 7,572 | 15% |
| 3 | California | 7,197 | 14.2% |
| 4 | New York | 3,925 | 8% |
| 5 | Illinois | 1,669 | 3.2% |

N = 50,797 (Total Active Latino Physicians)
SOURCE: 2021 State Physician Workforce Data Report, AAMC

population, Latinas/os are the country's largest racial/ethnic minority group, but they make up a far smaller portion of doctors.

According to the Association of American Medical Colleges (AAMC), Latinas/os comprise nearly 7 percent of all physicians in the nation. Most active Latina/o physicians are concentrated in California, Florida, and Texas, states that have large numbers of Latinas/os (table 1).[31] An even smaller share of US medical school faculty, only 3.2 percent, are Latina/o.[32] Why is their representation in medicine so low?

Olga hints at first-generation college student status as a launching point. We know that Latinas/os have historically occupied jobs on the bottom rungs of the occupational hierarchy due to race and class stratification in the United States. While some refer to this phenomenon as double jeopardy, triple oppression, or the simultaneity perspective,[33] others aptly suggest that the intersection of various factors determines their life chances and experiences in organizations. We also know that college-educated Latinas are concentrated in a limited set of female-dominated "semi-professions" and that K-12 education is the top occupation that they enter.[34] While they remain underrepresented in the better-paying, more prestigious occupations such as law and medicine,[35] they are making slight gains. Latinas, today, however, are more likely than their male counterparts to be in professional occupations, a complete reversal from prior occupational trends where men were more likely to be in managerial and professional jobs after the Civil Rights Movement of the 1960s.[36] Indeed, an early exploratory study on Latina medical students and doctors in the Los Angeles and Boston areas chronicled the multiple gender-related stressors women faced that began with gendered expectations in their immigrant families of origin, only to face others in the workforce.[37] When I asked her about her journey into medicine, Dr. Cecilia Paz, a sixty-two-year-old cardiologist of Mexican heritage, reflected, "It's basically a man's world . . . I've always dealt with this," noting the particular effects of gendered expectations that were ever present in her educational and career pathway as a 1.5 generation immigrant who was brought to the country by her parents as a toddler. She later experienced derogatory comments linked to ethnicity as a Latina doctor in ways different from Lorenzo's.

Gender and ethnicity intertwine and produce uneven weights among bilingual Latinos/as seeking "physicianhood" that shift over time. Because of the heterogeneity within the Latine population, they experience distinct types of oppression and opportunity when striving for, and while wearing, the white coat. This book addresses how these dynamic and shifting weights manifest for doctors and what this means for their practice. Naturally, Latina/o doctors today must also contend with these issues among Latine patients who come from diverse backgrounds.

## PAN-ETHNICITY AND HETEROGENEITY IN THE LATINE COMMUNITY

Pan-ethnic labels, of course, obscure heterogeneity within the group. Much as Rosa and Lorenzo differ in the gendered expectations in their families of origin, the Latina/o medical population consists of people with distinct migration and incorporation histories, holding different statuses under immigration policies, and are of a vast array of ethnicities and phenotypes. Language and immigrant generational levels produce a variety of outcomes for them in US institutions. While half of second-generation Latinas/os are Spanish/English bilingual,[38] the ability to articulate themselves in the Spanish language—an ethnic marker—largely unites them, and it is also used to demarcate social boundaries between them.[39] This book examines internal stratification and opportunities among Latina/o doctors in the US through their gendered narratives. Work in this area tends to emphasize intra-ethnic tensions between subgroups (Mexican vs. Puerto Rican or Cuban vs. Salvadoran) or moments of pan-ethnic solidarity.[40] Others focus on the important contributions of various Latina subgroups and the drawbacks of pan-ethnic labels.[41] Scholars note that the study of pan-ethnicity is focused on the "process of fusion as well as fission."[42] In contrast, I take an intra-Latina/o dynamics lens to examine how intragroup distinctions shape Latina/o physicians' experiences vis-à-vis their professional work demands as opposed to how they clash with other Latinas/os.

In disaggregating Latinidad, I find that Latina/o physicians' backgrounds are bifurcated; they either come from disadvantaged or unusually advantaged backgrounds. The AMA has influenced this by controlling the composition of the US medical workforce through educational entry requirements and immigration and governmental policies, especially via visa expansions, restrictions, and licensing laws. To be sure, racially biased performance metrics and hostile learning climates in US schools ultimately stunt the careers of all trainees of color, particularly those from backgrounds underrepresented in medicine (URM). These compounding disadvantages contribute to URM trainees' lower matching odds, steering them into less competitive and lucrative specialties, burnout, and attrition.[43] This racialized learning climate is crucial for doctors of color trained in US schools, who not only pay astronomical fees but often attend de facto segregated and underperforming schools. Significantly, many Latina/o physicians begin in the community college system, which some medical schools do not evaluate favorably.[44]

Latina/o doctors as a group provide a unique lens through which we can explore social mobility, race/ethnicity, and gender discrimination in American medicine. As a pan-ethnic group with wide-ranging characteristics, their ascribed demographic characteristics act like cumulative weights in their coat pockets, producing disadvantages for some and benefits for others. Most are US-born children of poor Latina/o immigrants who hold less than a high school education. Others are highly skilled immigrants who attained their medical degrees in Latin America, arrived as adults, and are considered international medical graduates.[45] Latin American IMGs entered the US with either an H-1B or J visa for highly skilled immigrants.[46] The number of H-1B visas is very small; applicants must meet several criteria, chief among them gaining entry into a residency program through which the visas are sponsored.[47] Recipients of J visas can avoid the normal two-year home residency requirement by working in federally designated Health Professional Shortage Areas or Medically Underserved Areas. The new doctor would have to show that they would experience persecution in their home country or that returning would bring exceptional hardship to the applicant's spouse and/or children who are US citizens or permanent residents. They could also try to obtain sponsorship by an Interested Governmental Agency.[48] Individual state health departments can also sponsor a maximum of thirty J-1 physicians each year, usually for practicing in underserved areas as well as under the Conrad 30 program.[49] All are sorely needed in hospitals and clinics that lack the infrastructure to provide care to a diversity of patients.[50]

The effects of colorism within Latinidad are important to consider, particularly in a US racial structure that operates under a rigid Black/white binary lens. The sociologist Ellis P. Monk suggests that a more thorough understanding of skin tone must consider how intragenerational processes of categorization fraught with skin tone biases produce cumulative benefits and costs via the body.[51] Latines run the gamut in phenotype from blond hair and blue eyes to black hair and brown eyes, and we know that among Latinas/os light skin is associated with higher earnings and more years of schooling attainment in the US.[52] Scholars who have examined the relationship between skin tone, discrimination, and internalized racism find that medium- and darker-skinned Latinas report higher discrimination at higher socioeconomic (SES) levels.[53] The lightest-skinned Latinas endorsed higher levels of internalized racism than all other skin shades. These results were gender-specific and were not observed among men. Skin color interacted with socioeconomic class status to predict internalized racism among Latinas. While skin color is often tied to racism and discrimination, race is not just about color but about the meanings and connotations that we apply and project onto people's bodies.[54] Some of the doctors in this book received their medical school training in the US and some in Latin America, regions with distinct racial/color classification systems.[55] I strive to capture Latina/o doctors' experiences of how people interpret human differences based on skin tone and nativity across a spectrum of gendered identities. There is a need to address phenotypicality bias in academic settings, a point this book suggests should be extended to the medical profession.

This book demonstrates some of the issues that we must address if we are to meet those needs. First-generation college students in the sample described applying and getting into medical school as bewildering, and structural discrimination did not cease to operate on them at any step in their education or careers. Instead, they quickly learned that the higher up they went in their field and the more experience they gained, the heavier the weight of disadvantage due to operating in a system designed to support non-Hispanic white and monolingual English-speaking men. The heaviest weights of all turned out to be the complex and cumulative weights of ethnicity, in particular linguistic capital and gender. Structural hardship comes not only from a complicated medical system but also from patients, nurses, other doctors, and structures of the job. Everyone is complicit in perpetuating this inequity. Linguistic capital results in unequal weights for Latina physicians who gain opportunities but are also over-included in labor tasks that other physicians who are not Spanish/English bilingual or bicultural cannot, or hesitate, to perform for their patients. Thus, while there is a veneer of equality that Latina/o physicians reach because they are economically well-off and hold a high social status, the intersecting identities of gender, immigration status, language, and phenotype continue to shape their professional lives. In line with intersectionality theory, it is bilingual and non-white-presenting Latinas who experience the lion's share of inequity in this masculinized occupation as they provide care to mostly co-ethnic communities that are extremely underserved and sorely desire their skills.

I explore multiple axes of stratification and opportunity that often influence work opportunities, constraints, and outcomes. To do so, I identify within-group patterns and how they reflect the larger structural forces that shape them. This allows me to assess internal stratification processes by dint of the intersection of social location markers such as gender, ethnicity, nativity, and phenotype in a profession that has white masculinist, gendered, and racial hierarchies firmly embedded within it and that favors English dominance.

## FEMINIST THEORIES AND RACIALIZED ORGANIZATIONS

Medical organizations and workplaces are neither gender nor race-neutral, even though there is a presumption that they are.[56] The medical profession is *both* a gendered and racialized organization in that it privileges men, whiteness, and heteropatriarchy—the assumption that heterosexuality and patriarchy are the default—in the US, but the inequities that manifest for non-white physicians are not always readily apparent. The sociologist Victor Ray shows us that larger racial schemas are connected to the apportioning of resources, habitual actions employees are expected to perform, and the racial tasks they are assigned in organizations.[57] Racial tasks, for example, are defined as "the work minorities do that is associated with their position in the organizational hierarchy and [that] reinforces whites' position of power within the workplace."[58] In the same vein, gender and work sociologist Joan Acker explains that all organizations have "inequality regimes" that serve to maintain and replicate larger patterns of gender and racial inequality.[59] Inequality regimes are fluid and can change depending on the group in question within the same racialized organization, such as medicine. The tasks that get assigned to specific groups provide sharp theoretical tools for analyzing workplace interactions and their connection to broader organizational hierarchies.

The gender discrimination and sexism that white women described in medicine due to its heteromasculine culture are redoubled and magnified for people who are not white. Education scholar Mia Ong notes that "to claim membership in science women of color must maintain the appearance of belonging to a culture of no culture."[60] For women of darker phenotypes, corporeal appearances stand at odds with the identity of STEM professionals, which requires them to engage in daily impression management strategies to communicate their expertise and competence in science. This comes at personal costs such as compromising one's identity. For women in science, elements of self-presentation include style and content of speech. Problems between social actors ensue when expectations over self-presentation clash. Such is the case in Kwon and Adams's assessment of Asian-Canadian women medical professionals in training who were advised by white women colleagues to remain "humble" to avoid negative interactions with nurses.[61] Other research, based on interviews with Black and Latina physicians, has noted that nurses were "more willing to serve and defer to male physicians," yet tended to approach female physicians as equals and were both "more comfortable and communicating with them . . . [and] more hostile toward them."[62] At the same time, women of color physicians received less assistance than their male colleagues with preparing equipment, finding case records, or organizing signed paper-work. Thus, nurses and coworkers perpetuated a discriminatory gender order and participated in the stratification of doctors.

The intersection of race and gender also leads to distinct workplace experiences for physicians of color. Race and occupations scholar Lata Murti, the daughter of a South Asian physician, explains that South Asian Indian physicians possess what she terms occupational citizenship—access to most of the same rights and privileges as whites only when perceived as being both professionally successful and eco-nomically beneficial to the US. Murti also uses the white coat as a meta-phor in her 2014 dissertation "With and Without the White Coat" to explain how elite South Asian Indian immigrant physicians are marked as occupational citizens during clinical interactions with patients when they are in the white coat. But outside of this context, and when they remove this protective garb, they are subject to racist treatment from colleagues, staff, health-care institutions, and the general public. The different forms of racism these doctors face, as well as how they inter-pret this racism, had as much to do with their gender, immigrant gen-eration, and perception of others' race and class, as with their professional class status. Moreover, gender and work sociologist Wasudha Bhatt explains that gender, race, and nativity status intersect to produce unequal experiences for South Asian women and men physicians who work in the US, with South Asian women doctors more likely to experi-ence sanctions for being brown or foreign-born in science than their male counterparts.[63] Like others before me, I also examine gender, eth-nicity, immigration status, and location of a medical degree, whether United States Medical Graduate (USMG) or International Medical Grad-uate (IMG), in workplaces.

Perceptions of race and gender discrimination in medicine also change depending on the social location of the group in question. When exam-ining perceptions of racial discrimination among Black doctors, sociolo-gists Adia Wingfield and Koji Chávez note that workers' experiences with racial and gender discrimination derived from their position within the organizational structure.[64] Black men physicians understood racism on the job as an aberration and indicated that racial discrimination was more likely to be experienced by Black health personnel who hold positions in the lower echelons of the medical hierarchy. Regardless of their position in organizational hierarchies, however, Black medical professionals experienced racial outsourcing, where they performed uncompensated equity work to make organizations more accommodating to minority patients.[65] In interviews with Latina/o doctors, however, I found that linguistic-based equity work leads to a range of inequality regimes that Latina/o doctors experience that are not solely determined by race but by gender, ethnicity, nationality, generation, socioeconomic status, age, and phenotype. Thus, Latina/o physicians' experiences with different forms of discrimination in medicine derive from intra-ethnic variation within the group rather than from their position within the organizational structure.

## LATINA/O PHYSICIANS AND THEIR STORIES

This book relies on seventy-four interviews with fully licensed self-identified and currently practicing Latina/o physicians—thirty-nine women and thirty-five men—and observations in their places of work between 2014 and 2023. This relatively long period allowed me to capture a cohort effect for those trained before and during the advent of increasing diversity, equity, and inclusion programs, Hispanic Serving Institution funding opportunities, as well as the COVID-19 pandemic. The fifteen interviews that took place between March 2020 and December 2020 occurred over the telecommunication platform Zoom. All of this is supplemented with secondary statistical data, an analysis of state trends, and research trips that exposed me to medical programs and scientists in Cuba, Puerto Rico, and Mexico. To be eligible for the study, participants had to self-identify as Latina/o and be a current practicing medical doctor or advanced intern. The doctors were practicing medical physicians or board-certified surgeons employed at hospitals, clinics, private practices, and medical groups all over California. I initially recruited them by contacting people with Spanish surnames on listed medical center department websites and emailing them an IRB–approved message. While this initial recruitment strategy did not include self-identified Latina/o physicians whose surnames are not in Spanish, most of my contacts referred me to all doctors in their network. This initial process led to snowball sampling, in which consenting physicians referred their colleagues and members of their medical school cohorts who were Latina/o, some of whom did not have Spanish surnames. A few physicians were also recruited after they gave keynote lectures at regional conferences hosted by Latina/o nonprofit organizations and online mentoring forums.

I also conducted interviews with twelve medical graduate students who technically have a white coat but are still in the early process of earning their degrees to practice unsupervised. Their narratives are also important for understanding pathways *into* the career, especially for a younger cohort of doctors who had diversity and inclusion programs available to them that physicians who attended medical school post-Civil Rights did not.

The interviews took place at a time and location most convenient to the doctors: private offices, hospitals, clinics, school campuses, and cafés or eateries during their lunch break. A twenty-five-minute interview with a male respondent was the shortest, with the longest reaching nearly three hours with a woman. Women were more generous with their time, indicative of the emotional labor they regularly expended. Ethnicity facilitated access as I traversed being both an "insider" and an "outsider" with physicians.[66] As the US-born daughter of Mexican immigrants who speaks Spanish more or less fluently, I found that they felt comfortable code-switching during the interviews with me. I was always attuned to different Spanish dialects. In many ways, I was an "insider" because I am a peer in a different high-status occupation and also a doctor. Yet, I was also an "outsider" as my social location did not fully emulate that of all respondents. I also do not possess a medical degree. All of the doctors, however, were enthusiastic about recounting their pathways into the occupation to help future doctor aspirants.

The interview guide included twenty-five open-ended questions that covered pathways into medicine, specialty selection, and "matching" processes, as well as relationships with patients, colleagues, and coworkers. Interviews were conducted in person and audio recorded unless the respondent preferred not to be recorded. In only one case, I took extensive notes and jottings during the interview because of such a preference, which I later turned into a lengthy memo. To protect participants' confidentiality, I gave them pseudonyms, and masked, or omitted personal details such as specialty where extraneous to understanding a theme or experience. At the end of the interview, all doctors were offered a $20 Starbucks gift card for their participation, which some declined. All the transcribed interviews were uploaded into MAXQDA, a qualitative coding software. As I coded the interviews for emergent themes I used a categorical complexity approach—a multigroup and comparative approach across configurations to obtain a "synthetic and holistic process that brings various pieces of the analysis together."[67]

## PHYSICIAN SAMPLE

Doctors I spoke with reflected the heterogeneity of the Latina/o population (see Appendix A). They identified as Mexican, Central American, South American, Puerto Rican, and Cuban. They also had varying degrees of Spanish language proficiency. Of the seventy-four respondents, fifty (68 percent) were of Mexican origin, which is the largest Latina/o subgroup in the US, and 83 percent of California's Latines (table 2).[68] Five were Central American (Salvadoran, Guatemalan, or

TABLE 2
Physician Ethnicity by Sex and Generational Level

| | 1st | 1.5 | 2nd | 3rd+ | Other | Total |
|---|---|---|---|---|---|---|
| **Female Ethnicity** | | | | | | |
| Mexican | - | 5 | 10 | 8 | - | 23 |
| Central American | - | 4 | - | - | - | 4 |
| South American | 7 | 1 | - | - | - | 8 |
| Caribbean | - | - | 1 | - | 3 | 4 |
| **Male Ethnicity** | | | | | | |
| Mexican | 2 | 2 | 21 | 2 | - | 27 |
| Central American | - | - | 1 | - | - | 1 |
| South American | 1 | 1 | 3 | - | - | 5 |
| Caribbean | - | - | 1 | - | 1 | 2 |
| **Total** | 10 | 13 | 37 | 10 | 4 | 74 |

Nicaraguan), thirteen were South American (Colombian, Ecuadorian, Peruvian, Argentinian, or Brazilian), four were Puerto Rican, and two were Cuban. Eight physicians who were born in South America, seven women and one man, had parents who worked in white-collar occupations such as physicians, engineers, educators, and lawyers in their home country. Ten were first-generation immigrants, meaning that they migrated or moved to the United States as highly skilled and multilingual professionals. Two physicians of Puerto Rican heritage obtained their medical schooling in Puerto Rico, which is considered a US medical school. However, two-thirds of the fifty Mexican-origin physicians had immigrant parents who worked in service or factory work. Almost 60 percent of them were the children of working-class immigrants, with thirteen brought to the US as children before the age of twelve and thirty-seven being the second generation and US-born. Ten were third or later generation and of Mexican heritage.

Nearly two-thirds of the doctors featured in this book had parents who did not attend college in the US or their country of origin. They were first-generation college students. Their parents worked in low-wage jobs such as gardeners, laundry pressers, fast food chains, or the garment industry. Women's ages ranged from twenty-nine to sixty-seven, and the median age was forty-three. Men's ages ranged from twenty-nine to seventy-six, and the average age was forty-one. Women on average had been working longer than men—fourteen years—while men had been practicing on average for ten years. Eight of the physicians were finalizing their medical residency programs and thus had lower salaries than the others but were on the cusp of transitioning into a higher-paid position. The rest were working for community clinics or larger medical organizations (some affiliated with universities) or had opened a private practice. About 51 percent of women worked in feminized specialties such as family medicine, obstetrics and gynecology, and pediatrics, mirroring the paths of women in medicine in general. In contrast, only about 30 percent of men worked in pediatrics or family medicine, and the rest in more "masculine" fields. Nine Mexican American physicians worked in a surgical capacity, with only two women in this category, an ophthalmologist and a cardiologist. The men worked as reconstructive, orthopedic, pediatric, general, or trauma surgeons. Surprisingly, over half of the sample (61 percent) specialized in primary care (family, internal or pediatric medicine). Two physicians described themselves as later generation and not Spanish proficient, but all others stated they were bilingual, although in some cases they overestimated their proficiency in medical Spanish. Men were more likely to claim fully bilingual capabilities, although my observations when we switched to Spanish was that they were less proficient than the women. Despite their lesser seniority, men, on average, earned much higher salaries than their women counterparts, with one earning well over $800,000 by virtue of large research grants. While most first-generation college student Latina/o doctors earned significantly more than their parents did, the wage gap was salient among women. "You have to keep fighting for your salary. . . . There is still bias even with salaries. Being a doctor, I have more money than my parents ever made. . . . [Y]ou know that other doctors, who are white men, are making more than you," remarked Dr. Olivia Martin, a Mexican heritage doctor in pediatrics. This was notably the case for Latina physicians who worked in academic units and were made aware of their lower pay when they were notified of equity salary adjustments by deans in their university systems after years on the job. Only three Latina doctors owned their practices. Five doctors declined to provide income information. While most were USMGs (US medical graduates), eleven were IMGs (international medical graduates).

On research trips, I spoke with physicians in other US states or countries in informal conversations, some of which I report here. For example, I met a Venezuelan family medicine doctor who worked at a large urgent care center during my visiting assistant professorship at the University of Hawai'i at Mānoa. He was an international medical graduate, having earned his medical degree in his home country, and then completed an internship and residency at a private elite university. I do not count these conversations with doctors in my overall sample, but they provide my study with a wide-ranging perspective. In the book's conclusion, I bring in a Cuban neonatologist I spoke with during a research trip with UC-Cuba to the island. This research trip exposed me to the medical system and many women STEM professionals there.[69] I dig deeper into this research trip in the concluding chapter to elucidate the drastic differences in gender composition in medicine between Cuba and the United States as a counterpoint to glean implications. The majority of Cuba's doctors are women, and the neonatologist's comments illuminated how gendered racism in the United States and the astronomical cost of higher education in America contribute to this unevenness.

## CLINICAL SHADOWING

I spent time in physicians' waiting rooms and offices, shadowing sixteen doctor-patient visits with fully registered medical practitioners.

These visits spanned from fifteen to sixty minutes. For all, the physician introduced me as a *doctora* or *profesora* and asked each patient if they consented to my being in the patient room. Only one patient declined to have me present. On some occasions, other students were training to become nurses or physicians. Other times it was just me, the physician, and the patient. I usually stood or sat in a corner of the office and took copious notes. I did not collect any identifying information from patients. Instead, I focused on how they described their ailments and how medical providers communicated with them and offered care. Like premedical students who seek shadowing opportunities, I signed an observer of care shadowing policy provided by the human resources department of a large HMO organization. I was also invited to medical galas/events geared toward fundraising scholarships for Latina/o students striving to attend postbaccalaureate programs. In all, I completed a total of fifty hours of observations.

Because the COVID-19 pandemic interrupted in-person observations in March 2020, I supplement the data in this book with formal coursework I undertook at an intensive medical Spanish program at El Instituto Cultural Oaxaca for one month in 2022. I took sociocultural health-related courses that train physicians, nurses, and those seeking health careers who wish to care for Spanish-speaking immigrant populations in the US and globally.[70] The program emphasizes the sociocultural and medical landscape in Mexico, which many migrants carry with them to America and California.[71] At the Instituto Cultural Oaxaca Spanish Language School, I learned medical terms related to human anatomy, symptoms of physical discomfort and disease, types and characteristics of disease, medical and surgical equipment, and how to approach and describe a patient.

To analyze doctor-patient interactions I borrow from one of the central tenets of critical race theory (CRT). This lens enables me to account for the role of racism and other forms of oppression in medical settings. I draw from two key race-related elements of CRT: 1) the centrality of race and racism and the intersection of other forms of oppression and 2) an emphasis on experiential knowledge. CRT focuses on both racism and intersectionality, a framework that investigates the ways that multiple marginalized identities interact with social hierarchies to shape individuals' lived experiences in multiple arenas and institutions.[72] Underscoring the experiential knowledge of patients is essential because a person's social location—identity categories that intersect and interact—shapes their everyday experiences. Further, Latina/o Critical Race Theory (LatCrit) scholars challenge the notion that Latine identity is essentialist; rather they argue that it is inclusive of ethnicity, language, nationalism, immigration, and residential status. Thus, CRT and LatCrit provide the tools necessary to analyze the experiential knowledge of patients and the linguistic capital of their providers.

## ANATOMY OF THE BOOK

In this volume, I put my finger on the pulse of the state of Latinas/os in US medicine and show how the weight of the white coat factors in different phases of their lives. Like a surgeon who carefully sutures an incision, I thread the needle through each chapter demonstrating how these context-contingent weights begin with the messages they received in their families of origin about their gendered career choices, then continued as they navigated STEM education and in organizations when caring for a diversity of patients as fully licensed practitioners. In chapter 2, I focus on the messages that Latinas/os received from their parents as they pursued careers in medicine. These context-contingent weights began in the home, especially for young Latinas who aspired to nontraditional careers. Men rarely received gendered messages about pursuing careers in medicine from their families, unlike their Latina counterparts. Chapter 3 provides the reader with a greater understanding of the circuitous pathways that these mostly first-generation Latina/o college students trudged. The weight of socioeconomic status and institutionalized racism illustrates the difficulty these doctors faced in meeting all of the requirements and ultimately practicing medicine unsupervised, which in many cases took longer than the conventional timeline. I contrast these experiences with those of elite IMGs who were able to enter the medical profession in a more straight-line fashion via opportunities embedded into institutions of higher education that are not readily accessible to poorer and minoritized physicians who are educated in American schools.

In that vein, chapter 4 shows how social capital networks become more consequential as aspiring Latina/o physicians move up the higher echelons of the educational hierarchy and through medical school into their *chosen* specialty. Mentors are the network hubs that could leverage their weight—connections, and reputations—to find aspiring Latinas/os health-related opportunities that otherwise would not exist for many of those who were first-generation college students. These significant others, however, exhibited different forms of support that influenced how Latina/o clinicians experienced training. In this early stage of their careers, bilingual Latinas interpret their linguistic abilities as an asset that provides them with a wealth of opportunities. I also elucidate how Latina/o physicians are channeled into primary care by various individuals and by graduate ethnic medical programs due to their gender and ethnicity. Chapter 5 captures how Latina/o doctors interpret other workplace actors' gendered displays of deference and demeanor toward them. We see the shift of the multivalent weight of the white coat as their bilingualism is no longer interpreted as an asset by organizational actors but rather a means of overinclusion in workplace tasks leading to exploitation. Ultimately, it is bilingual women who are tasked with performing the lion's share of Spanish language interpretations for patients. The intersection of gender and age also curiously shapes perceptions of authority and competence for them.

Of all the physicians that I interviewed, only one self-identified as Black Puerto Rican, but many were read as not entirely white. Chapter

6 shows how skin tone intersects with gender, class, and nativity and matters for stratification in medicine because it produces distinct status hierarchies for Latina/o medics, with white-presenting men doctors experiencing rewards and praise akin to what the white men who dominate medicine can expect. I illustrate how whiteness and masculinity are weighty organizational mainstays and determine opportunity structures and resource allocation in distinct ways for bilingual men and women doctors due to skin tone and physical attributes. The data in this chapter comes from interviews in which physicians shared their perceptions of how their phenotype impacted their experiences (or not) in the medical elite space. Relying on interactions between doctors and patients, chapter 7 of the book illuminates how Latina/o doctors are engaging in structurally competent care. This chapter shows how Latina/o providers "center the margins" by placing value on the knowledge and perspectives of their patients. I also show the emotional weight and toll that providing for poor Latina/o communities takes on doctors. I rely on ethnographic vignettes taken from doctor-patient interactions in distinct medical organizations. These vignettes are indicative of the types of linguistic and cultural interactions that emerge in medical organizations across the nation.

The conclusion provides a more global perspective. I concentrate on doctors who practice in California, but most had experiences obtaining schooling or training in other US states or abroad in other countries. My aim in using an intra-ethnic dynamics lens is not to highlight divisions within and among Latinas/os. Rather, I extrapolate how various patterns of inequality and privilege present in larger society interact and produce a conglomeration of outcomes for multilingual Latina/o doctors in one of the most prestigious fields around the globe. This book provides new theoretical and empirical tools and offers a more textured analysis of the various paths US- and foreign-trained Latina/o physicians take and examines what happens after that success has been attained. A major focus of social mobility scholars on middle-class minorities is examining the blocks to their vertical mobility within the job as they serve as the financial safety net for poorer family members. Moreover, work and occupation scholars are concerned with how patterns of inequality in larger society are replicated in jobs. I add to these frameworks by providing a holistic account of how Latina/o doctors who reach the end of the metaphorical "leaky pipeline" make it to the final destination of their journeys, and wrestle with continued micro-aggressions as they seek to do their jobs and provide care. The professionals I interviewed are extremely content with their choice to enter the elite medical profession and know they work in an occupation held in high regard. Their families are proud of them, too. Yet, for most, their achieved high occupational status only produces partial protection from gender and racial discrimination over those who more closely embody the demographic characteristics that medicine has privileged for decades. While there is a great need for more Latina/o physicians who possess linguistic capital, we cannot assume all of them will have the same challenges or opportunities.

Discrimination is not universal, then, but it is common. And it does not stop at the prohibitively high cost of entry. Even after earning their coveted golden ticket, bilingual Latinas/os quickly learned that some people within their ethnic group and some non-Latinos are already in the priority line. They quickly learned that providing culturally congruent care has a cost that is cumulative and produces uneven weights for them. Latina doctors who have linguistic capital may be the most sorely needed in medicine, but they also pay dramatic costs, costs that US society should begin to eliminate if we are to create equitable workplaces and health care for all.

# 2.

# GENDERED CAREER CHOICES

[My mom] opened a path for me for a life that she would have liked for herself. It was a paradox; she opened this path, but at the same time she resented me for taking it. It took me a long time to understand all of this, my mother's pain and frustration. . . . [My father] allowed me to dream, even though he didn't understand me, but I also felt so smothered. . . . I have a theory; I've asked the successful Latinas I know this question: Were you your father's favorite child? They all said yes! . . . There's something to that. Even if our fathers don't entirely understand us, being their favorite child somehow gives us this core of strength that helps us. . . .

—SANDRA CISNEROS[1]

GENDERED DYNAMICS WITHIN LATINE families are fraught with contradictions. The Latina physicians I spoke with reported experiences much like those of acclaimed Chicana novelist Sandra Cisneros regarding the varied reactions she received from her parents over the growing opportunities she was afforded as the daughter of immigrants and now a professional woman of color in the US. Tensions between gendered expectations for women from the immigrant parents' home country and those available in the host country were common as Latina physicians navigated their career choices in

Portions of this chapter are related to a previously published article: Flores, Glenda M. (2019), "Pursuing *Medicina* [Medicine]: Latina Physicians and Parental Messages on Gendered Career Choices," *Sex Roles* 81: 59–73.

America. Latina physicians born or raised in the US perceived their fathers' upbringing in Latin American societies as exhibiting patriarchal ideologies,[2] such as having decision-making power over women, yet they also perceived their fathers as seeing beyond such limitations for their daughters who were born or came of age in the US and had avenues to higher education. The Latina physicians I spoke with informed me that while their fathers witnessed and sometimes perpetuated gender subordination, they spared their daughters when it came to the pursuit of higher education and college degrees. They explained that their immigrant fathers often used the experiences of the poorer women in their lives, such as women relatives stuck with domineering husbands, to urge them forward in their medical studies. The conflicting messages of support and restraint that Latina physicians received from their parents regarding their medical career aspirations elucidate how changing structural contexts—such as access to higher education and entry into medicine—rearranged gendered ideals in their families in ways that their male counterparts did not narrate to the same degree.

In this chapter, I trace the messages that Latina physicians received from their parents about their gendered career choices into a nontraditional profession, and I selectively highlight a few narratives from their male counterparts to show the stark contrast in these recollections. As political scientist Maria Chávez explains, gendered inequalities and double standards that privilege sons in Latine families affect parenting practices and resources allotted to career selection.[3] The messages that Latino doctors received from parents pale in comparison to the contradicting messages Latinas received. These messages show men's privileged position in the family and society. In capturing recollections of how Latina doctors remember the parenting features of their upbringing I identify three primary patterns in these messages: (1) fathers' contradictory gendered expectations for their wives versus their US-born/raised daughters, (2) fathers and mothers' differing messages about procuring financial and social independence from men, and (3) parents' monitoring of their daughters' sexuality. In diagnosing these patterns, I argue that gendered ideologies applied to Latinas are rearranged not because of a modernizing Anglo influence or because their parents have adopted American norms, but because the cultural and structural landscape that these families have encountered shifted over time and has provided college-educated Latinas access to professions that were formerly only accessible to a white mainstream in America. For each gendered ideology, I use the recollections of a Latino doctor to exemplify how, unlike young Latinas aspiring to medical careers, male physicians seldom received gendered messages about gaining independence or had their sexuality monitored. These context contingent weights for Latinas aspiring toward the white coat began in the home.

## CONTRADICTORY GENDERED IDEOLOGIES

As the eldest girl in her family, Laura, a thirty-two-year-old family medicine doctor, described contradictory gendered ideologies within her working-class Mexican immigrant family. She described her father, from the central state of Jalisco, as "patriarchal" and the "man of the house," but also explained that he was progressive, "forward-thinking" and "astute" regarding the economic benefits a college education could reap for his US-born daughter. Laura's mother worked part-time in the cafeteria of an elementary school and was also primarily responsible for household duties such as cooking, cleaning, and rearing her two daughters. Laura's father worked as a gardener and was the main breadwinner. Laura explained, "My dad has two daughters, and he is very much, like, patriarchal. He is the head of the household, but I don't think it was ever an issue like 'You are a girl, you shouldn't think about [becoming a doctor].' If anything, he encouraged me." She shrugged her shoulders and smiled fondly. Such encouragement was typical of Latina physicians' fathers.[4]

Over half of the Latina/o physicians in the sample were 1.5 or second-generation and were raised by parents who held less than a high school education in their home country (table 3). A smaller percentage

TABLE 3
Highest Level of Parental Education by Latina/o Physicians' Generation, Status, and Sex

| Parental Education Level[a] | Female Physicians | Male Physicians | Total/Percent |
|---|---|---|---|
| **1st** | | | |
| <High School | - | 1 | 1 (1%) |
| High School Graduate | - | - | - |
| College Graduate | 7 | 2 | 9 (12%) |
| **1.5** | | | |
| <High School | 9 | 2 | 11 (15%) |
| High School Graduate | - | - | - |
| College Graduate | 1 | 1 | 2 (3%) |
| **2nd** | | | |
| <High School | 8 | 18 | 26 (35%) |
| High School Graduate | 2 | 2 | 4 (5%) |
| College Graduate | 1 | 6 | 7 (10%) |
| **3rd+** | | | |
| <High School | 1 | - | 1 (1%) |
| High School Graduate | 1 | 1 | 2 (3%) |
| College Graduate | 6 | 1 | 7 (10%) |
| **Other[b]** | | | |
| <High School | 1 | - | 1 (1%) |
| High School Graduate | - | - | - |
| College Graduate | 2 | 1 | 3 (4%) |
| n (%) | 39 (53%) | 35 (47%) | 74 (100%) |

[a] Parental education level is over-estimated. This table captures the highest level of education of one parent. The few parents who attained college degrees in the United States worked in education as teachers.

[b] "Other" includes parental education of Puerto Rican physician respondents.

of second or later-generation Latina/o doctors had at least one college-educated parent, most of whom worked in education-related spheres. The experiences of Ana, also in family medicine, show the tensions in some Latine families about pursuing the profession. She explained that her father, a Mexican immigrant who was raised in a small village in a central Mexican state, also expressed patriarchal ideals. Yet he openly shared how gender inequities impacted the well-being of his sisters and found it necessary to share this awareness with his daughters to prepare and push them forward. Ana shared:

[My parents] pushed the girls more. All of us have higher degrees than the boys [in our family]. . . . I asked [my father] a few months ago, 'Why did you want us all to be professionals? You come from a place where there is a lot of *machismo* and the women are expected to have babies and stay home.' He said, 'I didn't think it was fair.' He is close to his older sister, and she had a horrible life and a bad husband. She got married young, had a lot of babies, and was a housewife. . . . He didn't want that for his daughters.

By contrast, while Ana's mother was generally supportive of her aspirations, she was concerned that the length of time that medical training requires would postpone marriage and children too long. As Ana said about her mother's messages, "She was like, 'Why don't you choose something else? . . . A shorter career?'" Ana's parents had less than a middle school education in their home country and found themselves working as a landscaper and in a factory in the city of Santa Ana, a predominantly Mexican and Central American immigrant city in Orange County, where they settled. Past research suggests that migration from Mexico to the US alters gendered expectations and relations between Mexican men and their wives due to differing structural conditions in the host society but does not address the impact on the children of immigrants or parental expectations.[5] Recent work by Chicana/Latina feminists suggests that the bicultural daughters of Latine working-class immigrants routinely grapple with gendered cultural tightropes suffused with the ideals of *familismo* due to their parents' precarious socioeconomic position.[6] These are gendered cultural expectations that are associated with their ethnicity. The narratives from Latina physicians reveal that fathers espoused selective gendered ideologies for their upwardly mobile daughters as they pursued medicine and that this had profound impacts on their trajectories.

Janet, the US-born daughter of Mexican immigrants and currently a family medicine physician in her early thirties, described an even sharper split between her parents. She relayed that her devout Catholic mother "wasn't very supportive [of my career aspirations]. She was more like, 'Just go to church. Do a quick little college thing.'" By contrast, she continued, her father "definitely wanted me to be a doctor, surgeon specifically. My mom, she didn't. She wanted anything that would get me in and out of school the fastest." In some instances, mothers advised their daughters to select careers that required less schooling. This difference is in line with sociologist Jessica Vasquez-Tokos's findings among a sample of Mexican women who associated their national-origin group with oppressive gendered dynamics.[7] She found that wives who had to submit to gendered rules most strictly policed and tested other women, including those within their central and extended family unit.

However, Luisa, the eldest and only girl in her working-class and Mexican immigrant family, referenced strong support for her aspirations from her father in particular. She felt that her parents' relationship was quite patriarchal, but she described her father as "atypical" because he did not exhibit gendered ideas imbued with patriarchal notions regarding her future potential. She explained:

> [My father] always encouraged me. I don't think it mattered to him that I was not a son but a daughter. He didn't care about that. He knew he wanted something better [for me]. . . . There came a time when he wasn't able to help me with homework and school-related academics, but the moral support was there 150 percent.

Luisa felt that her parents' experience of having been pushed out of school at an early age to work in their hometown in Mexico and help their parents financially support younger siblings had motivated her father's ambition for her. She also felt that being the eldest in her family may have played a role in his emotional support. She attributed much of her success to the fact that her father pushed her as much as her younger brothers, implying some men with sons would not have treated their daughters this way. Luisa's account of her father contrasts with those of sociologists Ruth Enid Zambrana and Sylvia Hurtado, who found that Mexican immigrant fathers had high expectations for their daughters but were not always emotionally expressive in their support due to economic hardships and fears over their ability to help them pay for school.[8] Luisa's father's avid support, despite his low earnings working in a paint factory, is illustrative of his faith that his economic hardship and lack of a college degree would not serve as a structural constraint for his daughter.

Similarly, both of Vicki's parents encouraged her and her sisters to be ambitious. Vicki was a family medicine doctor and the US-born daughter of immigrants who were born in Mexico City. Her mother was a homemaker, and her father worked as a machinist. About the different messages she received from her parents, she shared:

> It was different. Both of them encouraged us to do well in school. . . . My mom was always more of the type [to say,] "do whatever makes you happy". . . . My dad encouraged us more like, 'I want you to be a professional.' I think it was always encouragement from both, but I think my dad won. . . . [He] grew up in Mexico City. . . . My dad was very poor growing up. . . . [He] remembers getting on the metros and selling gum on the street at the age of nine. . . . He didn't want that to happen to us.

While Vicki noted that both of her parents expressed their support for her schooling, her father was more explicit about the type of profession that he wanted his daughter to obtain. Her mother, on the other hand, focused more on feelings of contentment or the home because that was the limited option she was given. Moreover, while her mother gave a similar encouraging message as her father, Vicki recalled that her dad "won."

It was typical for Latina physicians to assess their educational and employment aspirations through the messages they received from their fathers about the less-educated women in their lives. This was also the case for those who were raised in middle-class homes with at least one college-educated parent. Nancy, a self-identified Chicana who grew up in an affluent Tejano family, felt that her parents' educational attainment differences were advantageous to her. "[My dad] is a veterinarian. I think he thought [family] medicine was a good career for me to choose. Financially stable. He always encouraged me to study. My mom not so much." Nancy explained that her mother did not finish college and found work in the education sphere in South Texas. For this reason, she felt that her US-born mother of Mexican heritage encouraged her to explore, have fun, and not work so hard. Dominican sociologist Nancy López notes that the daughters of Dominican, Haitian, and West Indian immigrant mothers on the East Coast assessed their educational opportunities against the backdrop of their mothers' hardships.[9] However, I find that most Latina physicians assessed their educational and employment aspirations through the messages they received from their immigrant fathers about the immigrant women in their lives who never had the privilege of pursuing education beyond primary and middle school.

Men, on the other hand, rarely received these forms of gendered career-oriented messages from their parents. All interviews that were with 1.5- or second-generation men who were raised in working-class homes reflected this. Benito is typical: the US-born son of Mexican immigrant parents and current family medicine doctor, he described his parents as equally supportive of both him and his older sister and their aspirations. His parents were from rural villages in Jalisco and Zacatecas. Benito's sister Ema was the first in the family to enroll in the University of California system, and he said that his parents were supportive of her decision to attend in Irvine, even though it was some distance away from their home in Pomona (about an hour's drive without traffic). Both siblings took a somewhat roundabout path to their professions. Ema majored in biology and had considered medicine but did not like her experiences in the laboratory and ultimately ended up getting her master's in teaching. She now works as a first-grade teacher in Pomona in a Spanish immersion and transition school. Benito agreed to the interview because he wanted to ask me about my first book *Latina Teachers* (2017). When I told him that several of the women I interviewed who had pursued or obtained bachelor's degrees in STEM were socially channeled into the teaching profession, he said that it sounded "true to form," as this description reminded him of his sister, but he felt the channeling had come purely from sources other than their parents. Initially, Benito had considered becoming an architect and was offered a full ride to a top architectural school.[10] Instead, he "followed [his] elder sister" to UC Irvine as she served as an important conduit of information for him. Ultimately, it was Benito who went to medical school. His words further show that his sister ceased to pursue medicine due to unfavorable on-the-ground experiences in science laboratories and not due to limitations imposed by their working-class parents.

## Gendered Messages Among Central and South American Women

Like their Mexican peers, Latina physicians from Central and South American families also described the fluidity of gendered processes in interactions with their fathers, some of whom possessed college degrees in their countries of origin. Lisa, a family medicine doctor, recounted that her father was very supportive of her career choice, but that her experiences in childhood reflected highly gendered divisions of labor. She had been born in El Salvador and moved to the US with her family when she was a year old. They settled in the Pico-Union District near downtown Los Angeles. Her parents were highly educated and had financially comfortable professions in El Salvador as a teacher and a university employee, but the government blacklisted Lisa's father for being an educator and the family fled, in fear for their lives.[11] They experienced downward mobility upon US arrival, a not-uncommon experience for Latin American immigrants.[12] Ultimately Lisa's parents found work in the garment industry, making neckties as undocumented workers. Lisa explained that when she grew up in the urban streets of downtown Los Angeles, in keeping with "a traditional role" she would "be the one cleaning the kitchen every day," and otherwise helping her mother with household tasks. Her brother, on the other hand, had minimal responsibilities, "to vacuum on a weekend or something." Lisa asked her parents to let her "switch roles" with her brother, to reverse the gender-based division of labor in the household. She explained that she would be the one to "fix cars" and "put up the Christmas lights with [her] dad," tasks that she deemed as gendered male. But Lisa indicated that her father did not limit or confine her career choices: "My dad was OK with whatever [profession] I did."

Claudia was also a family medicine physician and the daughter of Salvadoran immigrants who described a mixed experience in terms of her father's ambitions for her. Claudia explained that her father, who unlike Lisa's had struggled financially before migration, was "very conservative in El Salvador." At one point in her life, he had told her, "No, you're going to get married, and you're gonna have kids. You're not gonna have a career. You're a girl." Claudia said that her mother had wanted to get a job to alleviate the family's poverty, but her father would not let her: "My dad told [my mom] that she wasn't gonna work—that she was going to stay home and have babies." However, Claudia noticed that his expectations changed over time as she advanced in her studies at the University of California, Davis. She remarked, "I don't know if this idea is true anymore because when I was applying to college, I was like, 'Oh I think I'm going to do biology and be pre-med' and he was supportive. . . . When I came back from college in December one time, his gift to me was a stethoscope and a blood pressure cuff." Thus, time in America and access to higher education changed his outlook for his daughter.

Similarly to women physicians of Mexican and Central American origin in the study, South American physicians like Gloria, the daughter of educated Argentinian immigrants[13] who were exiled from the country when she was in high school, also faced these gendered contradictions in America. She noted, "Going away from your house to college is easier to let a young man do versus a young woman. There is still a lot around the importance of family and motherhood, which can be seen as being at odds with a professional full-time career like medicine." Gloria finished high school in America, and as the daughter of college-educated immigrants in a new country, she still encountered gendered cultural tightropes from her parents as she adjusted to US higher educational institutions.

In contrast to Gloria, however, physicians of South American heritage in my sample were more likely to have completed their medical education in Latin America and migrated to the United States when they were older (see chapter 3). Seven women physicians (see table 3)—all South American—had at least one parent who was a college graduate. It is striking that it was mostly foreign-born Latinas who sought opportunities to transition into American medicine, suggesting a potential lack of vertical advancement for women in science industries in Latin America as opposed to men. These women also generally had the support of their parents and especially their fathers for their career aspirations. Elsa grew up in a middle-class home with highly educated parents in Colombia. She had completed all her schooling in South America and moved to the US in 2001 to get more training and conduct research. She said, of her parents' feelings about both her and her sisters' careers, "My father is amazingly pro-female, because of men from his generation . . . there were more female-oriented professions, but my parents were not—whatever you wanted to study, do it well." Elsa's two sisters worked in the traditionally male professions of engineer and architect in Colombia. Thus, Elsa explained that her father, who was a professional in her country of origin, took an active role in her educational life and did not confine her to a feminized job. This is not to suggest that affluent Latin American fathers were less patriarchal than those who were working class, but rather that socioeconomic background and regional context are salient in gendered career selection.

In the same vein, Jazmín, a dermatologist of Colombian origins, also felt that her father was more supportive of her ambitions because her mother rarely provided her with a concrete direction. "My dad was more a big influence in the sense that he wanted me to be a doctor. . . . My mom never encouraged us, that's true. When I was going to apply for vet school or medical school [my father, an accountant] would always say, 'medical school is better, [please like that career].'" Even though Jazmín's mother was a physician in Colombia, she left her career to raise her children.

Whereas some Latina physicians noted that their mothers were initially not as enthusiastic about their career ambitions as their fathers, in other families both mothers and fathers were eager for their daughters to obtain financial and social independence to escape the limitations of patriarchy.

## PROCURING FINANCIAL AND SOCIAL INDEPENDENCE FROM MEN

On the day of the interview, Enrique, a pediatrician of Mexican and German heritage who self-identified as Chicano, was wearing cream-colored jeans, a black sweatshirt, a black beanie, and a pair of sneakers that did not match—one shoe was white and the other black. He had an ear piercing and a big wedding ring. His parents were from a rural town in Jeréz, Zacatecas, located in central Mexico. He recalled how the women in his life, his mother especially, doted on him while he was pursuing his medical training and living at home. As he leaned back in his swivel chair with his hands clasped behind his head, Enrique said,

> For residency, I lived at home. . . . Within our culture we do that; it is no big deal, and it's true. My mom baked for me every time I was on call. . . . I told my mom, 'I'm staying here until I get married.' And my parents knew that I was helping contribute to the family because I was making some money. But I'm like, 'I have a great thing going [here]. Why am I gonna leave this?' . . . I know I had it very good. Bless my mom.

Enrique's words underscore that he was making small monetary contributions to his family while pursuing his medical studies. Indeed, other Latino physicians worried about being familial financial providers. But men's contributions to the family were more about securing social mobility for themselves for their presumed future families. Notably, Enrique joked that he allowed his mother to continue caring for him, presumably until he married his wife to take up those responsibilities, further reproducing hetero-patriarchal ideals.[14] This dynamic is referred to as "gendered familism" by sociologist Sarah Ovink, where college-educated Latinos/as provide divergent interpretations of what a college education will bestow in terms of autonomy.[15] Men's autonomy was regarded as automatic, meaning that they did not attribute their independence to obtaining higher education. Latinas, on the other hand, interpreted gaining a higher education differently. Unlike their male counterparts, Latina doctors navigated a series of pressures from parents to succeed both educationally and financially at an elevated rate to procure financial and social independence from men.

Thalia explained the gender-biased double standard she witnessed:

> The challenges we [Latinas] have to endure. . . . We're not going to get pregnant, we're not going to use up the scholarship money, [our parents] have to believe in our word that we're committed [to educational achievement]. My goodness, they tire us! We are anchored to our families. They would never do that to a boy, *'Ay mi hijito vete, no te preocupes, yo te cocino, yo te visto, yo te arreglo'* [My son, go, don't worry, I'll cook for you, I'll dress you, I'll fix it].

Here, Thalia references what Maria Chávez calls the *"mi pobre hijo"* or "golden child" syndrome that hampers men and hurts both men and women in the family in different ways.[16] Unlike her three brothers, Thalia noted that she had to reassure her family that she was not going to waste the scholarship money she was awarded by getting pregnant. The comfort that a man like Enrique experienced at home in part relied on not being pressed about his sexual activity.

Latina physicians raised by immigrant mothers explained that they were initially conflicted about the prospect of their daughters moving away from their homes to pursue their studies,[17] much like the Asian Indian women who were encouraged to attend local colleges by their families.[18] In most cases mothers wanted their daughters to remain close to home, and in others, their daughters devised ways to maintain regular contact despite geographic separation. While several Latina physicians said they wanted to live at home and commute, others expressed that they commuted daily to attend medical school because their mothers did not "want them to leave the house," especially because they were significant to fulfilling familial obligations.

Sociologist Sarah Ovink's study of the college-going behaviors of Latinos/as who were raised in immigrant and working-class families found that gender predicted their understanding of what a college education would confer on them in terms of autonomy and independence. Men expected to be autonomous in adulthood even without a college degree, whereas women felt they might not be independent unless they obtained one. For Latino men, the focus shifted from "present to future family," meaning that men's discourse and behaviors celebrated individualistic spending with the expectation that the benefits of their educational labors would be reserved for their *future* families.[19] Though many Latinos and Latinas agree with familistic *attitudes* and highlight the importance of supporting the family, Latinas' behaviors more often demonstrated the provision of material and financial support for families of origin. All twenty-three of my interviews with 1.5 and second-generation Mexican and Central American men mirrored Ovink's findings. Latina doctors navigated a series of exigencies from parents to succeed both educationally and financially to secure their financial and social independence from potential romantic partners at a much higher rate than Latino doctors. Latina physicians expressed that both their mothers *and* fathers stressed financial and social independence, but for different reasons.

Latina physicians did not perceive that their fathers constrained their career choices by relying on traditional gendered rules in the same ways that mothers did. Vicki remarked, "My dad always made sure that we [his daughters] never depended on anybody else. . . . He definitely wanted to make sure that we always had money to buy food and have a house where we could live even if we didn't have a partner." Vicki attributed these desires to the fact that her father's sisters did not fare too well with their husbands, and he did not want the same fate to befall his educated daughter. I suggest that fathers' push or advocacy for their daughters to reach their career goals is a form of patriarchal protection. Sociologist Nancy López argues that US-born Caribbean women develop home-grown feminism from observing the struggles their immigrant mothers endured at home and in low-wage work sectors,[20] and here we see that Latina physicians draw from fathers' gendered career messaging too.

Yvette, a doctor in pediatric medicine and the US-born daughter of two Mexican immigrants, narrated that her father told her it was only through education that she "could be on [her] own" and not beholden to an unfit partner. Her father had worked as a line cook for a casino in Commerce, CA, and her mother for a Fortune 100 factory assembling home appliances. They both wanted better for Yvette and her brother. She described her mother telling her, "You and your brother are going to be working in some air-conditioned office somewhere and get to have nice cars . . . not sweating so much." Similarly, her father told her:

> When you grow up you're going to go to college and you're going to be somebody in life. You're not going to be working in the kitchens. Kitchens are so hot, *mija!* . . . It's like hell. . . . They were both kind of pushing my brother and me. There is no option; you're going to end up going to college. There's no, I can't, or I don't want to.

Because fathers understood that immigrants and lower-educated women in their lives did not have complete independence or "better" opportunities, they rallied their US-educated daughters for more.

Some Latina doctors explained that they were determined to be financially independent and sought well-paying careers to avoid their mother's fate. Elivet, the US-born daughter of Mexican immigrants and a family medicine doctor, said that her father was not a good husband; he was unfaithful and often absent. She had to rely on an extended male relative to drive her to Pomona College to turn in her medical school application to meet an approaching deadline because her father was not present to drive her. She was determined to be financially and socially independent from any man. Overcome with emotion, she told me:

> I always wanted to have a career where I could be independent because my father cheated on my mother. . . . I once asked why she didn't leave him. She said, 'What was I gonna do with my three girls?' She only went to third grade and she was a homemaker when she got married. So, she's like, 'I didn't have many options.' I didn't want that.

Elivet's experience is similar to that of US-born Caribbean women who observed the struggles their immigrant mothers endured at home. They saw them toil and in low-wage work sectors and aspired for well-paying careers. Elivet's father encouraged his daughters to get an education, and in some ways was more financially ambitious for Elivet than she was for herself. She had chosen to work in a marginalized community instead of maximizing her earning potential as her father had wanted.[21]

Elivet explained that her father migrated to the US at the age of twelve and worked extremely hard to move his way up in his job, ultimately becoming the owner of a nightclub. This success seemed to shape his capitalistic ambitions for Elivet. She said that he continuously made it "clear" that he wanted all his daughters to get an education and that he pushed her to think about the entrepreneurial side of the job when she was in medical school, pushing her to open up a private practice in a wealthy Los Angeles area. "My dad asked me, *¿No quieres estar en una clínica en Beverly Hills?* [Don't you want to be in a clinic in Beverly Hills?] Don't you wanna become like a business owner? Open your own clinic?'" she recalled. In her study of fatherhood, Gloria González-López observes that Mexican immigrant men embrace distinct social norms based on the gender inequalities they experienced before migrating.[22] Elivet's father conforms to this observation in that he pushes his daughter to pursue and seize newfound opportunities in the United States. His words also demonstrate how the expectations for his daughters are different from those for his wife, and how he did not want his daughter to lose out on advancement opportunities. His economic position within the family also gave him a gender advantage over her mother who had limited options, illustrating the patriarchal privileges he wanted to keep.

In contrast, Yvette, a doctor in pediatric medicine, and the US-born daughter of two Mexican immigrants, explained that both of her parents supported her medical-school aspirations but her aunts, and her mother's sisters, often questioned her career choice. She explained:

> [My aunts] would say, 'Why is she still studying? . . . Why isn't she married?' There was a lot of looking down upon my parents and on me because I wasn't married. . . . My parents are traditional, but my extended family is very traditional. I was a single female, living on my own—when I was in medical school, I had a one-bedroom apartment. My mom never told any of my *tías* [aunts] that I lived by myself because that is scandalous because they would've said, 'Why is she living by herself? She should be at home.'

To women's family members, this choice meant that they had to move away for school and forgo starting a family for several years, failing to fulfill heteronormative gendered cultural scripts. Yvette moved from her parents' house in Orange County to be nearer to an elite medical school in Los Angeles. While it may appear that Yvette was not constrained, that she relayed that her mother did not discuss her living situation with her sisters indicates that it was a concern. Like sociologist Jessica Vasquez-Tokos, I found that some girls were negatively evaluated by extended family members and were constrained by their gendered rules.[23]

Indeed, Karen, a family medicine physician, did not reference her parents as being concerned about her having a bad marriage, but they did interpret her career choice as implying she would never marry because she would still be in school in the period when they would have expected her to do so. Her father accepted the situation. She was the eldest and the only girl in her immigrant family, and at the time of the interview she was married. She explained that her parents did not understand why she had to attend undergraduate school for four years and then graduate school for four more. She said:

> My dad was like, 'Okay, you can never get married, because if you're in school you can't get married and be in school.' So that was a dilemma for him, but I told him it's been hard for me to get to where I am, so it is unlikely for me to throw it away for a husband or boyfriend. . . . To [my parents] [marriage and school are] mutually exclusive, specifically because we are older by the time we get into medical school.

Vicki explained that she saw similar patterns among the Latina medical residents she was currently monitoring and mentoring, specifically resistance and concern from their mothers. In some cases, parental pressures to be financially independent consisted of discouraging them from pursuing a profession that takes a long time to degree. They favored quicker options. Vicki did not experience this herself, as both of her parents had been supportive, but she said that the Latina medical residents she was currently monitoring and mentoring often described resistance and concern from their mothers. "Their mom says, 'You're gonna regret it.' Or [their mothers are] in financial need and they say like, 'You need to go to work and start making money.'" Such messages align with other research showing that Latina/o children are expected to contribute to the household both financially and socially at much younger ages than other young adults.[24]

Another reason participants' parents want their daughters to succeed on their paths toward the white coat is due to what Rob C. Smith calls the immigrant bargain,[25] and this may explain why most parents encouraged their daughters to pursue medicine despite the time it takes. Immigrant parents sacrifice and toil in socially demeaning jobs so that their kids can study and get ahead and work in offices. About her degree, Yvette remarked, "It's my mom's degree, it's my brother's degree, and it's my dad's degree because all three of them made their own personal sacrifices to get me to where I am today." Janet said that her parents were sensitive to the prestige attached to the white coat, that they enjoy boasting *"Mija la doctora"* [My daughter the doctor].[26] Thus, both fathers *and* mothers professed financial and social independence for their daughters to escape the limitations of patriarchy. The sense that their daughters should access a non-traditional occupation to combat an unfair gender order added to the immigrant bargain, and fathers tended to be more concerned about how their daughters could leverage their careers in an attempt to offset gender disadvantage in the long run.

## SEXUAL POLICING AND MONITORING

The mothers of many Latina doctors in the study policed and monitored their daughters' sexuality. Among the men doctors, Alejandro, a thirty-five-year-old Mexican American internal medicine doctor practicing in Salinas, California, had initially left home at his parents' request that he monitor his sister, who was away at college, on their behalf. Alejandro said that his parents boasted regularly about their doctor children; his sister was an optometrist. Alejandro explained that his parents had less than a sixth-grade education and that they grew up in the jungles of the Mexican state of Colima near Minatitlán. Alejandro recounted that "he wasn't the best student" initially and his younger sister "lapped him" and was admitted to UC Berkeley via a California Promise Scholarship that she attained for her academic achievement in community college.[27] He had attended community college too but had been admitted to UC Riverside without a scholarship because his grade point average was too low. Worried about his ability to pay for school, Alejandro explained that his mother came up with an innovative plan. His mother told him to move to Berkeley and get a job and "*Ya puedes cuidar a tu hermana* [Now, you can take care of your sister]," he said, mimicking his mother's voice and chuckled. Full of glee about this newfound opportunity that required him to work and make sure his sister was solely focusing on her studies he remarked, "Cool, that's my job?" Alejandro happily obliged. Meanwhile "my sister was pissed" at the arrangement, he said as he laughed. He took pre-medical courses at a local community college while living in Berkeley. He ultimately gained entrance into the university and went on to medical school, but he never received any messages linking moving away for school to his sexuality from his parents. Rather, he was encouraged to move to chaperone his sister.

There is an assumption that immigrant families with similar conservative/traditional gendered expectations respond in the same way when confronted with new structural contexts, such as when immigrant families settle in urban neighborhoods or women have access to higher education. Immigrant fathers helped their aspiring physician daughters prepare for the move away from home for school, while some of their immigrant mothers were initially aggrieved about the process but came around after. When Vicki applied to a four-year university her mother did not "want her to go far from home" because she was worried about her daughter's safety and sexual activity. Her father, on the other hand, "was okay with it. He wasn't sad. He just said, 'If [going to a distant school] helps you concentrate on your school [that's good]. . . . Let us know what you need. We'll go take it to you during the weekend.'" Her father's statement that they would make the drive to bring her anything she needed was indicative of his support of her decision to live on campus.

Feminist Gloria González-López explains that the Mexican men she interviewed in Latin America perceived the cities they migrate to and the immigrant barrios where they settle as sexually dangerous for their daughters.[28] Latina physicians explained they allayed their fathers' worries about their sexuality by emphasizing that they were focused on the economic gains a professional degree would confer to the family. Karen's parents had warned her that having a sex life could derail her ambitions. They told her that "a lot of girls in the United States get pregnant at fifteen. A lot of them got boyfriends and didn't make it out of high school." She reassured her parents that she had worked too hard for her ambitions to "throw it away" for a man.

While fathers were supportive in general, they did not hesitate to address sexuality more or less directly. This contrasts with the findings of other scholars who suggest that mothers and daughters communicate more frequently over sexual issues than fathers and daughters.[29] Many Latina physicians found themselves negotiating moving away for school with their fathers by emphasizing the long-term financial security their eventual career would provide the family. Those who pursued their medical residencies away from home shared that their father's involvement in their education was often conveyed through messages about trust. For example, Luisa explained that her father "let her" move away for school because he trusted that she was going to prioritize her studies. It did not matter to him that she was a woman, and he went "out of his way" to drive her to conferences and anything school-related. She recalled that he had allowed her to attend a leadership program in Washington, DC, that lasted five weeks when she was fifteen. "I think that is almost unheard of [in Latine families]. He also had full trust in me [when I went to UC Davis for college]." Luisa's father also accompanied her on the Greyhound bus to universities outside of their hometown such as in the Sacramento area because he was excited about the selection process and wanted to ensure her safety in new surroundings.

Similarly, Thalia, the US-born daughter of Mexican immigrants who settled in a predominantly Mexican and Central American immigrant city in Orange County, explained,

> [I had to tell my] family, if you don't let [me] go [I] won't succeed because you are keeping me, holding on to me. . . . My dad would say, 'Lo voy a creer cuando lo vea' [I'll believe it when I see it]. Not that he was being mean or anything, but me being a girl, a woman. That's not what we did. So, no salgas con tu domingo siete! [Don't come back pregnant!][30]

Thalia had become a doctor of internal medicine. Her statement "That's not what we did" meant that young women in her family did not move out of the house for a prospective career unless they were married. She reasoned with her father, and he allowed it, but with reservations. In many ways, the strict social control that Latinas were subjected to had a positive influence on their education; it propelled them into academic achievements, as other feminists of color have argued, for example with regard to young Vietnamese American women.[31]

Elivet's mother also expressed concern about her daughter moving away for medical school. The furthest school Elivet applied to was in San Francisco, but in the end she remained close to Los Angeles to be near her ailing mother who was diagnosed with breast cancer. Elivet explained that her mother admonished her not to be sexually active in college even though she was no longer living in her parents' home. Her mother's words were etched in her memory: "[My mom said] nobody's gonna want you if you slept around kinda thing. I got all that. I got all the *'pórtate bien'* [behave] and we would talk almost every day! . . . I knew she was worried that I wasn't behaving." Elivet said that her mother was "worried. *'¿Qué vas a ser de libertad allí? . . . La vida libre?'* [Are you going to be [sexually] liberal there? The free life?] You're gonna be sleeping around and you're going to get knocked up. And you're not gonna be a good wife, or a good kid."

The stories of these women align with those of other researchers who find that immigrant parents strongly police the sexual morality of their daughters.[32] Sociologist Nancy López notes, "Among women, the intention to delay marriage and child-rearing was always discursively linked to the stigmatization of their sexuality and the importance of acquiring educational credentials for dismantling those stereotypes."[33] Certainly, these Latina doctors were aware of the dominant representations of Latinas as hyperfertile and wanted to subvert that stereotype via entry into a high-skill career. My findings do not entirely align with others' that Mexican women are more likely than Mexican men to be concerned about their daughters' sexuality, reflecting internalized sexism and the wish to protect their daughters from material consequences of female sexuality that they observed in the home country.[34] While the Chicana feminist scholar Gloria Anzaldúa indicates, "Males make the rules and laws; women transmit them,"[35] fathers were more likely to be concerned about protecting their daughters from sexual danger in urban city centers and ensuring their daughters' socioeconomic advancement rather than about preserving their daughters' virginity per se. Unlike mothers, who were worried about their sexual activity in school which would violate cultural norms, fathers were more concerned that daughters would return with an unplanned pregnancy that might derail their efforts to finish their medical schooling after so many years of dedication. Latina physicians were counseled by their fathers to obtain a prestigious career to escape patriarchal gendered experiences.

## GENDER, SOCIAL MOBILITY, AND TIME

Of the women physicians in the sample who attained their schooling in the US, only five moved to another state (Nebraska, Massachusetts, New York) for their medical school training. A few of these women were third- and fourth-generation. Esther, a self-identified Mexican American OBGYN physician who was fourth-generation, gave "credit" to her US-born and single Mexican-origin mother for encouraging her to move away from home to pursue her collegiate studies in medicine. Esther explained, "[My mother] was like, 'Go! Leave now!' [laughs]. . . . She let me go." Colleagues of hers who were the US-born children of immigrants, on the other hand, had a different experience:

> A lot of my [Latina] friends—like, their parents wanted to hold them back. They wanted their children to stay local and not to go out of state. . . . [My mom] had to raise us on her own. . . . It wasn't traditional for us like mom stays home and dad works. . . . I think that helped her to let me go off. The majority of my friends stayed home. One, they couldn't afford [to live off-campus]. And two, they preferred to stay closer.

In contrast to most first-generation college Latinas who were raised by immigrant parents with low levels of education, Esther's mother was a teacher, and most later-generation Latina physicians also had mothers who were college-educated.

The gendered ideologies Latina doctors encountered in their families are not static; instead, they evolve. Sociologists Eddie Telles and Vilma Ortiz note that "traditional gender attitudes lessen with generation since immigration and from parents to the children."[36] Traditional (or transitional) gender ideologies persist in the second generation among the US-born children of immigrants, but may change in subsequent generations.[37] The fact that Latina doctors entered a career not traditionally female seemed to have facilitated this process. That is, it is not just generation but *career selection* that challenges gendered ideologies in Latine families.

Likewise, Rocío explained that her US-born and college-educated mother was the one who "had to go out of her world to go to college," indicating that her mother bore the brunt of gendered strains in her immigrant family when attending college. In my previous study of Latina teachers I found that Latina daughters with middle-class mothers who had a career, even in traditionally feminized jobs, were more likely to escape traditional gendered attitudes in the home but not at work, as they were still subject to gendered biases.[38] A recent study of Latinas in doctoral programs highlights that they experience what the authors term gendered cultural tightropes.[39] These gendered cultural tightropes—imbued with the ideals of *familismo*—are experienced by all Latinas in academia, independent of class and immigrant generational level, because of the social categories they inhabit in white, individualist institutions. Martha, a third-generation Mexican-origin physician in pediatric critical care, explained that her mother worked as a teacher and her father as a principal while raising their seven children in Texas. Unlike the majority of Mexican-heritage women physicians in the sample who were raised in immigrant and working-class families, both of Martha's parents were college-educated. She explained that she grew up "upper-class" by Texas standards but would be "upper-middle-class in California" because of the higher cost of living. Her siblings had occupations such as electrical engineer, teacher, dentist, and musician. Being the sixth child meant that her older siblings were also able to guide her and open up pathways that they had already successfully navigated both in school and within the family. She explained, "I lived with two of my best friends away from campus. My parents were okay with it because my other siblings had done that." In effect, siblings, especially elder siblings who had navigated higher education, were able to set the example and guide younger ones. While the daughters of Latine working-class immigrant parents grappled more intensely with gendered cultural tightropes due to their parents' precarious socioeconomic position, even those who were raised in affluent homes narrated that their families could not help them navigate gender discrimination and inequities in their workplaces.

Gendered norms and attitudes toward sexuality change over time and over generations for women who enter white-collar fields. While some scholars have assumed that Latine parents all subscribe to conservative or traditional gender ideologies and socialize daughters in similar ways, changing structural contexts challenge monolithic and static ideals of Latine family dynamics. The narratives of Latina physicians reveal that fathers espoused selective gendered ideologies for their upwardly mobile daughters, although not for women in general. Unlike some immigrant mothers who had lower levels of education and were more concerned with the material consequences attributed to sexual activity in their home country, fathers were more concerned about their daughters jeopardizing the completion of their professional career trajectories in pursuit of the white coat. Fathers' messaging, in particular, indicate their strong belief that a nontraditional career in medicine could help their daughters achieve gender parity. Through Latina physicians' retroactive recollections, I find that some immigrant fathers want to maintain their patriarchal privileges for themselves, and yet seek patriarchal protection and the best possible life course trajectory for their daughters. Part of the reason they do this is because of the love they have for their daughters, but it is also because gendered expectations for women in the home country and those in the US are markedly different. This tilts the balance scale for the daughters of immigrants, adding a weight to the pan that their male counterparts rarely share. Gloria González-López broadens our understanding of Latino fatherhood as exclusively, *machista*, dominant, and authoritative, writing, "Fatherhood may become a family emotional process, through which men may begin to resolve and disrupt family patterns that promote gender inequality as they educate a new generation of Mexican American women with regard to sexuality."[40] I find this was also the case for parents who hailed from other countries in Latin America, such as Colombia and El Salvador. Contradictions in gendered ideologies can be explained through the desires that fathers of various national origins and class backgrounds had for their daughters—wanting financial and social independence from men for their daughters, yet also strategically professing sexual moderation as they moved through the educational hierarchy because they wanted them to ensure their professional goals as doctors. The narratives of Benito, Enrique, and Alejandro all bolster and reflect the contradictions in these gendered dynamics in that parents rarely professed sexual moderation in the pursuit of their careers. An intra-Latine dynamics lens shows us that gendered dynamics in the home produce uneven weights for first-generation college-educated Latina doctors.

In their narratives Latina physicians demonstrate that these gendered ideologies are rearranged not because of a modernizing Anglo influence or the acculturation process. Rather the cultural and structural landscape that these families confront has shifted over time and has given these women pathways to careers that were previously only available to white men. Later-generation Latina physicians with college-educated mothers were more able to escape some of these gendered rules as their career ambitions afforded them some freedom relative to their mothers and aunts. Yet, while Latina physicians have non-traditional careers, they are in many ways tied to gendered scripts in their families of origin, despite gaining structural access to higher education and the professional workplace. Even though their families hope that a career in medicine will protect them from gender subordination, Latinas are still subject to gendered biases embedded in American institutions of higher education and workplaces independent of their generational level or socioeconomic class status. Nevertheless, medical schools should factor in gendered dynamics in the home into their admissions and retention process.

In the next chapter, I explore what it takes to become a physician in the United States, and the distinct challenges that both poor first-generation college-educated Latinas/os and elite international medical graduate students navigate when seeking occupational entry.

# 3.

# CIRCUITOUS PATHWAYS

"I WAS JUST LOST" is the phrase that all first-generation college Latina/o US medical graduates (USMGs) conveyed to me about their meandering roads into medicine.[1] Because they lacked the financial capital and resources of affluent, white, or international medical graduates,[2] Latina/o physicians who were first-generation college students—that is, no parent or legal guardian earned a four-year college degree in the US or abroad—experienced circuitous paths into medicine, often characterized by significant delays. While their end goals were clear, as first-generation college students they had significant trouble figuring out what the pathway to becoming a medical doctor looked like due to fundamental institutional failures in serving students and professionals in this underserved group. In this chapter, I argue that socioeconomic status and the anemic efforts to address institutionalized discrimination in higher education gave rise to the circuitous pathways into medicine for poorer and first-generation college Latina/o doctors who attended American educational institutions (USMGs). I use an intra-Latina/o dynamics lens to bring to light the institutionalized racism that Latina/o USMGs had to navigate at the everyday level in colleges. Latina/o USMGs who were first-generation college students mostly came from working-class families who needed their help and could not offer them financial support, held precarious legal statuses, faced blatant racial discrimination in the US educational and medical school system, and possessed lower levels of cultural capital than their Latin American international medical graduate (IMG) peers. A look within Latinidad allows us to see that positively selected Latin American IMGs bypassed these forms of discrimination. In what follows, I detail what it takes to become a physician, and I end the chapter with narratives from the IMGs for contrast to bolster the discrepancy in the weight of structural discrimination in STEM education in America.

## THE BARRIERS LEADING TO CIRCUITOUS ROUTES

Gaining admission into medical school requires a long course of study, usually four years of college. Students may have any major but those who major in a science-related field have an advantage, and all must complete pre-med requirements. Every medical school has its own specific set of prerequisite courses, and these may change occasionally, but they usually require successful completion of courses related to biology, chemistry, organic chemistry, and physics (trigonometry or calculus-based).[3] Other courses vary and may be in disciplines like psychology, sociology, statistics, philosophy, or the humanities. All but six of the seventy-four Latina/o physicians I interviewed majored in STEM-related fields, most in biology and physiological science, but some began their trajectories in history, social welfare, interdisciplinary studies, Spanish, American Studies, Chicano/Latino Studies, zoology, and public health. Two of the twelve medical graduate students I interviewed majored in anthropology and social welfare and education as undergrads, while the rest majored in biology.[4] (Appendix B provides details on these participants.)

Majoring in biology or a related science discipline had the advantage of offering students priority access to the courses that were necessary for medical school. However, some of the Latina/o doctors and medical students I interviewed noted the hardships they faced in these courses due to the subpar preparation they received in their poorly funded K-12 schools that were mostly focused on getting them to master the English language and had limited science courses.[5] Several of those who majored in STEM fields at the outset of college experienced an unwelcoming atmosphere, academic probation, pressure to select another major, and the risk of losing financial aid.[6] These were profoundly upsetting experiences. Karen, who was the daughter of working-class Mexican immigrants and is now a doctor in family medicine, noted, "You go from getting straight A's [in high school] without effort to realizing you need to learn how to study in college. . . . I did pretty badly in my first quarter at UC San Diego. I was a biology major. I remember failing one test in chemistry and I had to drop the class. I didn't fail the class, but I did withdraw and that put me behind." These setbacks and a sense of playing "catch-up" in the sciences and biology was a common distressing narrative among US-trained Latina/o doctors. Regardless of their majors, the pressure to obtain good grades in their science courses to gain admission to medical school weighed heavily upon them, especially as they considered that most institutions relied solely on academic metrics in their admissions process.[7] To be sure, American medical schools have been characterized as racialized organizations that reproduce class and racial inequalities, rather than dismantle them.

These sentiments were echoed by Jennifer, a second-year in medical school at the time of the interview. Jennifer was brought to the US by her Mexican immigrant parents when she was an infant and she attended public schools in the San Diego region, near the border. She recalled that when she started college at UC San Diego, she was one of several

Latinas in her undergraduate housing hall planning to major in biology. At the end of the school year, she realized that many of her friends had already transitioned out of the major. She had to persist on academic probation and take a series of pre-general chemistry courses during the summer after her first year to pull herself out of academic probation and better prepare before enrolling in chemistry courses. She recounted:

> Bio was kicking my butt. I loved the classes, but I just couldn't get an A or a B. I was always getting a C or a C+, and I just could not hang—I did not know the foundations. I knew a little bit but not enough to get me through. What helped me have a good foundation, and then do well throughout G-Chem [general chemistry] [was the summer course]. I was considering changing my major to chemistry and then O-Chem [organic chemistry] happened. I was like, "Holy crap, I can't do this." At some point in my second year, I got put on academic probation because I had a few C minuses that had pulled my overall GPA [down]. . . . I was on that cutting block of, 'Am I going to get thrown out of this major?' A lot of my friends had by the second biology class in their first year, gotten kicked out of their major.

Latina/o USMGs who were first-generation college students recounted similar experiences at research-focused four-year universities.

Figures 1 and 2 show the retention and attrition rates of Latina/o students who began as biology majors in the 2010 and 2011 academic years. I collected this secondary data from a large public research-intensive university and used these academic years because they allowed me to track student trajectories longitudinally, assess what their pathways were, and approximate how many of them earned a medical degree. Both figures show proportional relationships. There were more young women in the sample (F = 326; M = 206), reflective of their higher enrollment rates in four-year colleges overall. From figure 1 we can gather that out of one hundred undergraduate Latinas who began as biology majors, only twenty-nine graduated with a Bachelor of Science.

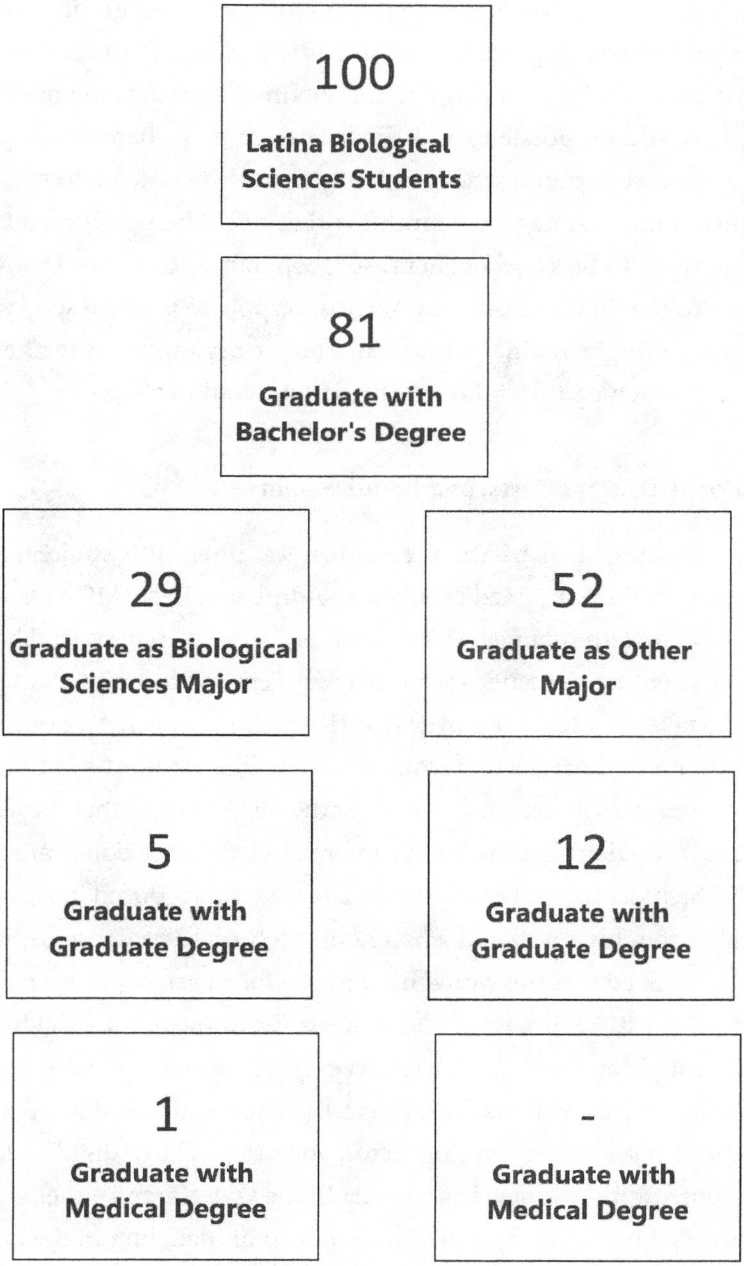

**Figure 1.** The Latina Undergraduate Student to Medical Degree Pipeline. Source: Author's own research.

While eighty-one Latinas that began as biology majors graduated with a four-year college degree, about half of them switched to another non-STEM major, and out of those none obtained a medical degree, even though would be possible, as I show later in this chapter. Only one Latina (and five men) who originally enrolled as a biology major obtained a medical degree. Jennifer is that one. She persevered and is now on track to become a general surgeon, but it took significant persistence to obtain the classes she needed to apply to medical school. She credited joining a Latina/o medical student organization for helping her persevere, a pattern I discuss in greater detail in chapter 4.

## Additional Testing, Costs, and Requirements

Upon obtaining their baccalaureate degrees, pre-health students must also score well on the Medical College Admission Test (MCAT), which evaluates problem-solving, critical thinking, written analysis, and knowledge of scientific concepts and principles. Fees for those in the United States to take the MCAT are over $300.[8] Raquel, a Mexican American physician in internal medicine, recounted, "The biggest hurdle is trying to get into medical school. . . . Can you get the MCAT scores that they want? Because if you don't get the MCAT [score], *les vales* [they don't care about you]." The most recent version of the exam was introduced in April 2015 and takes roughly seven and a half hours to complete.[9] Karen explained that she realized that she would need to pay for a prep course to help her study. "The MCAT is a whole other beast [from the SAT]. I did have to take it a couple of times. I took a ten-week [preparatory] course. My scores went up immensely. If you don't take the course, if you don't pay that $1,500, which is another limiting factor, you are at a huge disadvantage. I had to borrow [the money] from my dad," she said. Karen's father worked at a factory, but he saved up the funds to help his daughter in the pursuit of her medical dream. Like Karen, several Latina/o physicians took the MCAT more than once to try and improve their chances of admission.

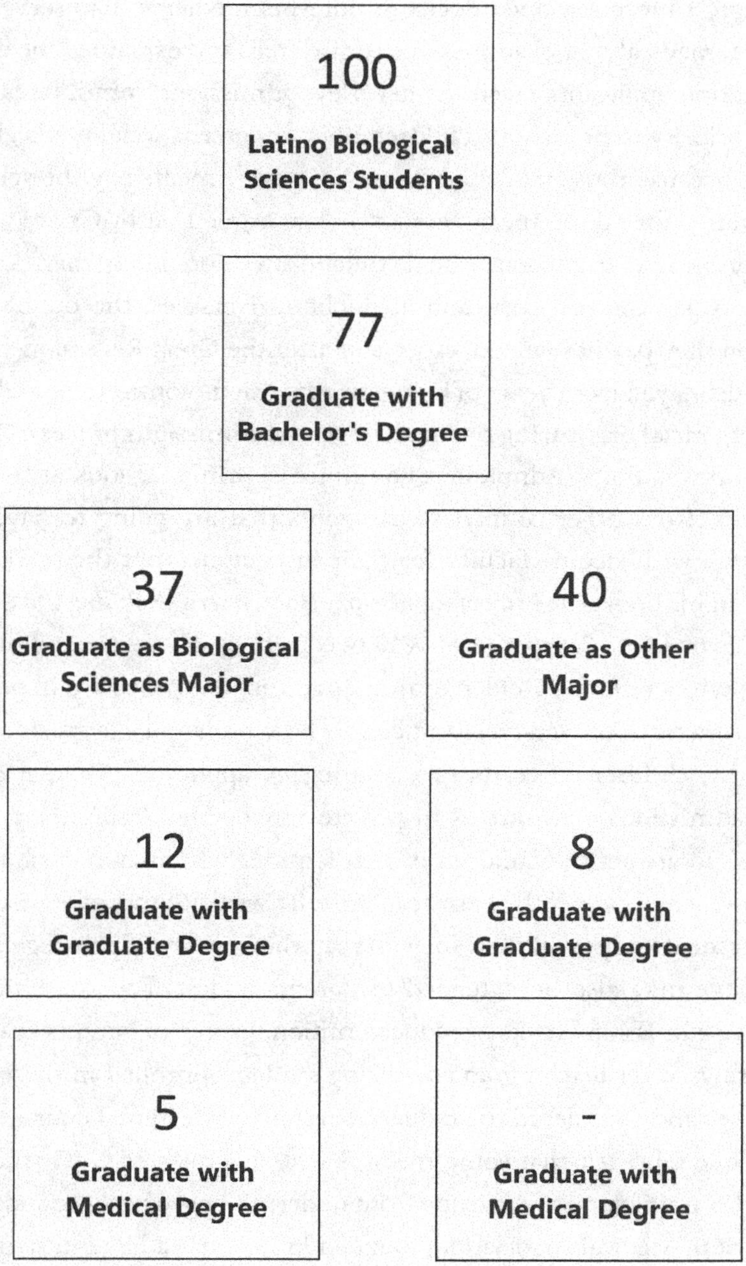

**Figure 2**. The Latino Undergraduate Student to Medical Degree Pipeline. Source: Author's own research.

Olga, a more seasoned doctor in internal medicine, had served on several medical school admissions committees and explained the barriers Latine applicants faced. In her view admissions committees first gave priority to professors' children, then to international medical students because those students' countries' governments pay the schools premiums for taking them. Some scholars argue that IMGs are at the end of the line, but international students are more likely than Americans to pay the full cost, and at public universities, the out-of-state tuition they pay has helped, especially after the Great Recession.[10] Possibly dismayed from years of being on admissions committees and witnessing racial bias during the medical school admissions process, Olga's opinion was that "[Admissions committees] primarily look at the top doctors [from other countries], as people that are going to have the research and become faculty for their institutions, not the [US] Latinos." In his book *The Price of Admission: How America's Ruling Class Buys Its Way into Elite Colleges—and Who Gets Left Outside the Gates,* Pulitzer Prize winner Daniel Golden examines admissions processes in private elite American universities, and details how preference is given to the wealthy, children of celebrities, and legacy applicants. Golden notes that admissions committees in private universities "relax their standards" to attract the children of rich families who may contribute to endowments, even if they are academically weak. Some, of course, are not academically weak, but they all reap the benefits of privilege. This privilege may also be extended to parents and staff whose children receive admission breaks or reduced tuition. Professor parents saw this as a reward for teaching and servicing students enrolled in these universities and considered the reduced tuition a professional courtesy.

While Olga felt that some medical schools preferred IMG students over US-trained ones who came from underprivileged backgrounds, the American Medical Association, founded in 1847, has a hand in structuring this. For example, the AMA historically regulated when "qualified" women physicians and Black doctors could join the organization, and at one point, in 1938, required that all foreign-trained physicians obtain citizenship status to regulate the influx of IMGs.[11] This rule remained intact for many state licensing boards until the 1960s, when a mass shortage of physicians in the US prompted the government to implement a "special skills exception" to attract international medical graduates to work in low-income and marginalized communities. IMGs are not a homogeneous group, and medical sociologist Rebecca Schut finds that those trained in developed countries such as the United Kingdom, Sweden, or Spain face fewer disadvantages relative to IMGs from developing countries (such as Mexico, Colombia, or Brazil) in their US careers.[12] Indeed, most Latin American IMGs in my sample were positively selected and possessed the human, social, and financial capital to move. They often worked alongside Latina/o USMGs, but Latina/o USMGs like Olga adopted a substitutionary, rather than a complementary to USMGs, lens.

In all, the estimated costs to gain entry to medical school can exceed $10,000,[13] a reason some Latina/o doctors experienced delays in their trajectories as they tried to accumulate the funds to financially smooth their paths while also trying to contribute economically to their poorer family members.[14] Primary and secondary application fees[15] also presented hardship. Medical admissions committees review applications and then invite candidates they might admit for in-person interviews with an admission panel, and candidates must pay their travel costs. Some interviewees explained that they applied for a credit card to buy interview attire. Karen explained how difficult it would have been for her parents to help her with these costs: "My parents were poor. We survived with $13,000 a year for a family of five." Evaluators who take part in these medical school interviews attempt to gather non-academic information that cannot be assessed via other means, such as a candidate's staying power, coping skills, interpersonal relationships, commitment to minority communities, and compelling personal characteristics like the difficult-to-measure altruism. Up to eighty-seven different qualities may be assessed depending on the programs available at each institution.[16] One study employing mock medical school interviews found that lower-income prospective Latine medical school applicants with family incomes of less than or equal to $20,000 scored lower than others in the sample.[17] This disparity became evident when Cecilia explained some of the mistakes she saw medical school applicants make in front of the admissions panel. When Cecilia would ask students, "Why do you want to be a doctor?" they would respond, "I want to help people." "Duh! That's stupid," Cecilia said. Cecilia reminisced about her interview: "I didn't let them speak. They just listened to me. I went in and said, 'I want to be a cardiologist because cardiovascular disease is the number one killer in the country. I want to use electrocardiograms.'" Because Cecilia had served on admissions committees, she knew the responses they favored and acknowledged that some Latine candidates were unaware of these higher-scoring responses. This is how racial bias manifests in medical school admissions as those who reap the benefits of privilege have supports that can provide this crucial form of capital.[18]

Medical school typically lasts four years, with two years of coursework and two years of clinical rotations, where medical students deliver supervised care and learn about different specialties. In medical school, graduates must then "match" with a job to carry out their residency and to continue refining their specialty. This process is also very expensive. Lorenzo, who had citizenship status, shared that his undergraduate loans amounted to $17,000, but that they had mushroomed to $245,000 by the time he was done with medical school and his surgery specialization. "It's a mortgage," he said, noting that he would most likely be paying off his loans for the next couple of decades. Physicians from working-class backgrounds incur more debt than those from affluent families because they cannot readily rely on accumulated wealth and family financial support. Rafael, who was of Mexican heritage and undocumented when he began college, could not pay the $30,000 tuition. He grew up in a trailer park and a GoFundMe helped him raise $10,000 for medical school, but it was nowhere near enough. Legal status blocked his access to federal student loans and stipends for medical school.

The median amount of debt reported by medical school graduates was $200,000 in 2019.[19] Differences in education debt by medical student race and ethnicity are influenced by whether they attended private or public schools and how they funded it. The median debt for a Latino medical student is just shy of $190,000[20] compared with $200,000 for a white student and $180,000 for an Asian student. Black medical students accrue the highest median debt, at $230,000, because a higher percentage of them attend private medical schools.[21] Compared with all medical school graduates of 2020, Asian graduates were less likely to report having education debt despite attending private schools at a higher rate and were able to rely on familial financial support.[22] Roughly 75 percent of white graduates attending public medical schools reported having educational debt, but also had the highest median parental income at $150,000, and also reported they relied on parents, relatives, or partner funds to defray the cost. Black and Latino medical graduates were 91 percent and 84 percent more likely to accrue these astronomical figures, respectively. Of all racial and ethnic groups, Latinas/os reported the lowest median parental income, at $70,000,[23] and were more likely than all other groups to take out loans. These figures are also further stratified by ethnicity, with Dominican-heritage medical graduates reporting the lowest median parental income ($36,000) both among Latinos and among medical students overall.[24]

Aspiring physicians must also pass the rigorous United States Medical Licensing Exam (USMLE) before they are permitted to practice medicine unsupervised. This exam has two parts, clinical knowledge and clinical skills, and costs more than $2,500 to take. International medical graduates must also pass this examination before practicing in the United States unsupervised. They have the same training and examination requirements as USMGs. For first-generation college students of color educated in US schools, however, circuitous pathways were structured by constraints in families of origin and the communities where they lived.

## THE CUMULATIVE WEIGHT OF NOT HAVING
## A DOCTOR PARENT

When I asked Dr. Marisa Delgado if there were any other doctors in her immediate or extended family, she responded, "No. I think in Nicaragua? I've heard there's somebody that's a professional in the medical field. I don't know exactly. Other than my brother, nobody." Several Latina/o doctors who were USMGs had some sense that a distant relative had practiced some form of medicine in the home country, but it was not only unusual to have a doctor parent; most did not have aunts, uncles, cousins, or grandparents who had practiced medicine either. When education scholar Patricia Gándara examined the lives of low-income Mexican Americans who received doctoral, law, or medical degrees during the 1960s and 1970s, she found that quasi-legendary family stories of distant professional family members were important sources of cultural capital.[25] In line with these findings, most of the Latina/o USMG physicians I interviewed were first-generation college students from working-class homes, and hearing "lost fortune stories" was a means of establishing family worth despite demeaning or diminished circumstances in America. Rarely had they ever had contact with these illustrious family members in the homeland, but the tales remained as unconfirmed legends in their minds, and a hopeful possibility for them in the face of numerous challenges.

Unlike research on Black doctors and South Asian physicians,[26] I did not identify strong co-ethnic/co-racial role models in my interviewees' past. The doctors in their studies were mostly raised in middle-class homes with college-educated parents. They excelled in high school and college because they knew they would need top grades to navigate post-secondary school. All described encountering a Black or South Asian

Indian doctor in their formative years, either a parent, aunt, uncle, or grandparent, or a doctor they met because a relative was dealing with a chronic illness. These experiences contrasted with USMG Latina/o physicians, who like Rosa in chapter 1 recounted the pressures of serving as interpreters for relatives during doctors' visits, as the children of immigrants often do.[27] In some cases, they attributed their interest in the field to these brief encounters, but few were like Adia Wingfield's respondents in feeling strongly drawn to medicine from the age of five or younger, and such encounters did not offer support or cultural and social capital to help them navigate their higher educational journeys.

Marisa described her circuitous journey to medicine thus: "[M]y story is so like, choppy and patchy and non-traditional. . . . I got here with all the bumps and bruises along the way." Marisa's parents brought her to Hercules, a city in Northern California, when she was five years old in 1985. As undocumented Central Americans, the family arrived in the United States when Temporary Protected Status was not yet available to Nicaraguans.[28] Marisa graduated from high school too early to benefit from a 2001 California provision allowing undocumented residents of the state to pay in-state tuition at its colleges or Barack Obama's 2012 Deferred Action for Childhood Arrivals program.[29] She was ineligible for federal aid and faced difficulty finding supportive medical school programs. Marisa's brother Julio, now an internal medicine doctor, was born a couple of years after the family migrated. Julio, who I also interviewed, attended the same schools as his undocumented sister, as many children of mixed-status families do.[30] Yet, he experienced what sociologist Laura Enriquez calls "multigenerational punishment," the spillover effect of growing up in a mixed-status and undocumented family throughout his life.[31] Marisa explained that their family was undocumented for "like 25 years" and that the process was prolonged because their lawyers "lost paperwork multiple times." She described her family having "to resubmit and pay the application fee multiple times." Her mother kept meticulous records so that every time the paperwork was lost, as they waited to be helped by Ronald Reagan's Immigration Reform and Control Act (1986), she had it ready to send in again. "As long as we were pending, we were in this limbo." The family also struggled financially; Marisa and Julio's mother worked taking care of the elderly, but even after she gained certification as a nursing assistant her wages were low, and their father was an alcoholic who was not always present and worked in maintenance only intermittently.

This limbo had cumulative consequences for both Marisa and Julio as they navigated the higher education system while helping their struggling parents financially. Marisa and Julio attended school together in the Mission District, a neighborhood in San Francisco that was well known for its large Central American immigrant population. Marisa noticed the academic tracking in her high school early on, where students were grouped differently based on their performance. Because she was doing exceptionally well in her classes she was placed in the honors curriculum and told which courses to take by academic counselors. Academic counselors were mostly available to high achievers. This experience made her acutely aware of the disparities between her and her peers in "regular" classes. Marisa explained,

> I was put in honors courses and then suddenly there were no more Latinos there. [My peers] had recently immigrated so they didn't have the language, but they may have had the capability. . . . It was a poor school. I'm sure they didn't have enough [money] to have a bilingual teacher or offered classes that they can use to get ahead in English courses along with their math and science. [Other Latinos] were [taking] ESL all day, basically, instead of complementing or supplementing their studies with other [STEM-related] courses.

The situation Marisa describes is typical; urban public schools emphasize English language proficiency. High-stakes tests require this emphasis and do not test proficiency in science, engineering, or technology.[32] These subjects usually take a back seat in urban schools like the one that Marisa and Julio attended, affecting their ability to connect with STEM teachers or substantially gain exposure to the curriculum before enrolling in college.

Nevertheless, Marisa excelled in school and gained admission into several top universities. But because of the precarious "legal limbo" she was in she had to pay international student fees when she was trying to fulfill the requirements for her bachelor's degree in American Studies at UC Berkeley. "That's an extra $10,000 per semester that they tag onto your tuition because you're not a resident or a citizen, even though I had been here since I was five. I got my papers when I was 20, 22, and then [I had] to wait the five years of residency before [I could] become a citizen." Much like Rafael, who took a two-year break due to his legal status and couch-surfed for a while, both Marisa and Julio had to delay their schooling multiple times by taking leaves of absence to work so that their family could make ends meet. Marisa even put her parents' house in her name when she was in college, but it was foreclosed on in 2008 during the Great Recession and she had to drop out of college for a period. It took her about ten years to achieve her bachelor's degree. (It took Rafael six.) Whereas many candidates begin their journey into medical school in their early twenties, Marisa was not able to officially begin medical school until her late thirties.

The siblings felt the weight of socio-structural disadvantage and noticed the limitations of their cultural capital. Julio's temporary break from UC Berkeley not only pertained to his parents' financial need but also to a lack of mentors. He explained, "I dropped out not 'cause I wasn't smart enough, maybe because I thought I wasn't? . . . I didn't find the right mentor. [I] didn't know who to look for, what to look for." A parent or other elder who had gone through medical school would have been advantageous; as he recalled, he had at least ten classmates in medical school who were the child of at least one doctor (see chapter 4 for more on social networks). Marisa tried to help Julio, but she lacked a mentor as well. An American citizen for over a decade when we spoke, Marisa was still coping with the financial toll, legal ramifications, and length of time that pursuing medicine took on her and her family when she was a student.

Delays in schooling are all too common for upwardly mobile Latinas/os who are often the financial safety net for their families, where the flow of monetary support is often from children to parents instead of the other way around.[33] Dutiful daughters explain that this affects their career choices and they sometimes opt for white-collar fields that take a shorter time to degree. My previous work calls attention to the fact that many Latinas who enter teaching stay there. I found that those who had pursued degrees in STEM were socially channeled into the feminized teaching profession due to class ceilings in their families of origin. This almost became the reality for Dr. Lisa Macias, whose parents were educators in El Salvador, although their degrees were not recognized in the US. Unlike Rafael, Marisa, and Julio, Lisa had some cultural capital and entered the teaching profession to help defray some of the costs of medical school even though she had gained admission to a program in Southern California. Four years of undergrad, then four years of medical school, and then three or more years of residency were costly. She also factored in the time and the "breaks" she took to study for the MCAT or to save money. Having taken some education classes in undergrad, Lisa reasoned,

> The traditional [medical] student [applies] junior year [in undergrad]. It takes a year to apply and then when they graduate, they already have a position, and they go straight. I ended up taking six years off to study for the MCAT. I did not have enough money to pay for medical school, so I decided to teach for a little while and make some money.

The regulations to become a teacher changed soon after Lisa entered the field, and she took the appropriate tests to stay in the profession and formally obtain a teaching credential. The money she was making in her job and working in a lower-income school district allowed her to study for the MCAT and take a coupling course. This time around, she applied to twenty schools and gained admission to a prestigious program. Because of socioeconomic constraints in their families of origin, many first-generation college-educated Latinas sought out the quickest post-BA option to become financially solvent and help their struggling family members, and they remained teachers. Lisa, however, was one of the very few who transitioned out of teaching when she was able to dedicate herself fully to medical school.

## SURVIVING THE HIGHER EDUCATIONAL GAUNTLET
### Weeder Courses

STEM courses for first-year undergraduates are often called "weeder" or "gateway" classes because if students do not perform well in them, they will not be able to remain in the major. Some of these courses enrolled more than six hundred students who had minimal to no contact with the professor. It was incumbent upon them to develop relationships with teaching assistants, form small study groups with their peers, or try to learn the material on their own. Marisa described her experience in a famously difficult course:

> I tried taking organic chemistry. It was horrible. . . . I left my first exam crying and I cut that class out. 'What is this on this test? I've never seen this in my life!' You just don't have anyone to ask. Because I was undocumented, I didn't feel like I belonged there. I had huge impostor syndrome. I didn't feel like I [could] go into the office and say I need help or where can I get a tutor? It was almost like I was auditing the classes. . . . I would just show up and try to learn something, and I'd just go home. I was never part of the campus community, like organizations.

Being an undocumented student made Marisa feel isolated not only in her science classes but in the campus community overall.

Elivet, a family medicine physician whose father wanted her to open a private practice, described a similar experience of alienation with general science professors who taught in large lecture halls. "I didn't interact with [professors] much at all. I think I went to the office once because I was doing so bad, and I was figuring out how to fix it," she remarked. STEM courses are often described as having a chilly atmosphere, with gendered interactions in the classroom dissuading women from continuing.[34] Nancy, a doctor of family medicine, recalled, "People were weeded out; there were lots of people failing chemistry or not doing well. Not getting above a C in chemistry and therefore a lot ended up dropping out of the pre-med pathways back then because of that."

Men also recalled these experiences in college while on the pre-medical track. Thomas, a third-generation Mexican American and the first in his family to attend college, recalled the weeding-out process thus:

> Anywhere you go, UCLA, UC, Irvine, Berkeley, everybody's pre-med. That's what happened at UCLA when I first got there. Everybody was, 'Oh, yeah. I'm pre-med.' All these Latinos like, 'I'm pre-med.' Then all of a sudden, I was taking chemistry with them. They're dropping out like, 'Let's go somewhere else, get another major'. . . . All my friends that I knew at UCLA that were in their first year saying, 'I'm going to be a doctor' and ended up getting hammered in the first couple courses in sciences and they got weeded out. A bunch!

Latina/o physicians described these courses as brutal, competitive, and lonely. They felt they had to figure everything out on their own and could only approach faculty when they were in dire straits.

In contrast, Cynthia, an IMG in internal medicine who was trained in Perú, felt she had a more collective rather than individualistic and competitive experience in medical school. She tied this cutthroat mentality and culture in STEM to America's rugged individualism. About her schooling in Latin America, Cynthia relayed,

> In Latin America it is more collective . . . over there, everyone is, 'Come here! Look, I found this. Look at this on the microscope. I will let you use it.' We would share it. We all worked well together. Some

people knew more and that was okay—they knew more. I am not going to worry because they know more, or they scored higher than me. There wasn't that.

The competitiveness was also not as prominent as US-educated and trained physicians relayed about their experiences in large science classes. Cynthia continued,

> We studied not to be better than the other one. Not to win in grades with your classmates, not to crawl over each other in grades. I never felt that pressure in my university life. We studied because it was important to study and because we wanted to know and understand well enough so that at any given moment, we could put it into practice to benefit the health of the town.

Cynthia's description contrasts sharply with Latina/o USMGs' description of science courses as being run by the principle of "survival of the fittest," where only the strong survive. Latina/o doctors' main purpose in referencing Charles Darwin's biological theory of natural selection was to invoke a sense of brutal competition, but Cynthia's description suggests that there is another way. Instead of being designed to "weed out" students who are "not strong"—as the experiences of participants suggest, it eliminates students who might be strong but who have been underprepared by their high schools—courses could *strengthen* interested students and propel them toward success.

## MAJORING IN NON-STEM FIELDS

A few Latina/o physicians started as pre-med and opted for non-STEM disciplines. Esther, who was a fourth-generation Mexican American, completed her undergraduate schooling at a private research university in New York. She described how being a history major, even though she knew that she wanted to be pre-med, helped her to cope with the demands of STEM classes. Esther explained,

I knew that you didn't have to major in biology to go to med school. . . .
Science was hard for me. It was never easy. Calculus and physics?—I don't
think I could get a good GPA to get into medical school if I majored in
science because it was hardcore, chemistry and organic chemistry. I had
to work hard. I went to tutoring sessions. I went to study groups. I had
friends help me. I was taking courses to get into medical school. I was
doing that in the background. History was my major because I was good
at that. I was good at humanities. I was good at writing. It was harder to
work at sciences, so I think my third year at UCLA I was like, 'Well I have
all these sciences classes now, but I like history and I am applying to
medical school. I should just do two majors. Why not?' So, I did. At that
point, I applied for physiology as a major and got my BS. I spent five years
at UCLA. . . . I ended up doing an extra year to do all my sciences—to double major.

Double majoring added time to Esther's undergraduate experience,
but she strategized to maintain an adequate grade point average for
medical school.

Thomas also pointed out another advantage of combining a history
major with pre-med courses at UCLA, an emerging Hispanic Serving
Institution: he felt that it was valuable in equipping him to practice
medicine, even though it did not help him satisfy the prerequisites for
medical school. He said,

Number one you need your degree. Does it need to be in the sciences?
No, it doesn't. . . . A lot of people do physiology, biology, microbiology,
genetics [but] you can be a dance major and go into medicine. [I thought]
'What if I go into [general history] and I do pre-med at the same time?' In
medicine you need to talk to people, you get their history, you get to know
people, you get to know where they're from. . . . There's always communication. Science, math, history, everything is in medicine.

To do this, Thomas also had to be intentional and tailor his course
loads every quarter so he "had half history, half sciences." It is signifi-

cant that both Esther and Thomas were later-generation Mexican Americans, and had one college-educated parent (neither in medicine), signaling that they had acquired some cultural capital that others were still developing.

In contrast to Thomas and Esther, Ricardo, a first-generation college student, made a similar point at a public event geared toward Latina/o undergraduate students who were interested in pursuing careers in the health-care industry. Ricardo was asked to talk about how he was able to become a physician with a degree in Chicano/Latino Studies and how majoring in this field combined with his pre-medical and residency experience better prepared him for his job as a family medicine physician in marginalized and immigrant communities in the cities of Los Angeles and Santa Ana. He shared that he had taken Chicano/Latino Studies courses at East LA College and that he graduated with a degree in Chicano Studies from a prominent school. Ricardo explained that at UC Berkeley, an emerging Hispanic Serving Institution (HSI), it was possible for students to major in non-science fields and to also enroll in certain pre-med requirement courses. He also emphasized that Berkeley's strong ethnic-based program helped students enrolled in health careers:

> When I took my Chicano Studies course, I started . . . making the connections with health and thinking, 'This is me, this is my family; this is what we go through. Maybe I could be a doctor?' . . . [My brother] went to medical school and he dropped out. I ended up getting motivated, going back to school, taking all the science classes. . . . Once I did, I went to UC Berkeley, and [that grew] even more.

Latina/o physicians who were first-generation college students valued non-STEM courses for helping them to make connections between STEM and the social determinants of health in their communities, but it also added more time, in some cases many years, to their trajectories.

## OBTAINING PRE-HEALTH REQUIREMENTS OUTSIDE OF FOUR-YEAR COLLEGES OR POSTBACCALAUREATES

Community colleges are the main arterial pathway for Latine students into medicine. A recent national study helmed by Dr. Efrain Talamantes and colleagues found that one-third of first-year medical students begin their premedical undergraduate education at a community college or two-year college, and Latines had the largest representation.[35] The Talamantes study argues that community college attendance, however, is a negative predictor of acceptance to medical school. Participants' experiences complicate this data, as they report that STEM faculty in community colleges were highly supportive as they completed their pre-health requirements. By contrast, many ran into problems with faculty (or counselors) at four-year colleges who were overwhelmed with research demands. Ana, a forty-seven-year-old family medicine physician, described her pathway to medicine thus:

> I didn't do everything straight, directly. I went to Santa Ana College. I got my AA degree. Then I went to UCLA and got my bachelor's degree in physiology. In between there, I told myself if I can't get into medical school, I will get a master's in public health. But I got into medical school. I finished [my coursework] but I didn't go straight to residency because I was a little older and I wanted to settle down. While I did that [that is, got married] I went to Cal State Long Beach and got a master's in public health. Then I came back to residency.

For Ana, the whole path was demanding. In her point of view, the length of time was necessary for her to form a family[36]—a desire both she and her family had for her—and because she did not want to be in residency while showing signs of pregnancy to protect herself from gender bias.

Marisa attended various local community colleges to fulfill her pre-health requirements after earning her BA and before applying to medical school. As she said:

I took my courses at local junior colleges, and I made sure they were transferable to UC credit. I submitted five transcripts when I applied to medical school because all these schools had to give me credit that would add up to the prerequisites. I couldn't afford a postbacc [that is, a postbaccalaureate program designed to prepare students for medical school]. Usually, they're $20,000, or $30,000. I made up my own informal postbacc, and it took me five years to do what would usually take two years because I was working full-time, and I would just take one class at a time during my work.

Postbaccalaureate programs at both private and public universities are costly, as Marisa described, and range from $20,000 to $40,000 for one to two years of additional schooling. Other doctors also enrolled in postbaccalaureate programs to become stronger candidates for medical school. Mauricio, in critical care, explained that he did not have adequate mentorship—a pattern I touch on in greater detail in the following chapter—and "waited hours to see" the sole premedical adviser who was on his undergraduate campus to receive some advice. Because of this gap in mentorship, Mauricio was directed into a postbaccalaureate program. He explained,

When I was done [with undergrad], I said, 'Okay, now what? When do I take the MCAT? Where do I apply?' That's one of the reasons I got directed into a postbaccalaureate program. They prepare you, teach you everything, and make you into a strong candidate. It's an additional year but . . . I don't think I would be here today if I would have done it on my own.

Mauricio, the son of a landscaper and a housekeeper, demonstrates how his parents' lack of human capital affected his pathway in ways similar to Rosalva, the US-born daughter of poor Peruvian immigrants. Her parents worked in a cannery and as a dairy truck driver. Rosalva also enrolled in a dual MA in medical science/postbaccalaureate program to improve her performance in science-related courses before applying to medical schools. This added two more years to her journey.

Thus, Latina/o USMG pathways into American medicine contrasted significantly from elite Latin American IMGs and those who were raised by a doctor parent.

## "I DON'T FIT THE TRADITIONAL [LATINA/O USMG] NARRATIVE": HAVING A DOCTOR PARENT

The most linear and direct route into medicine takes ten to fourteen years from the start of the undergraduate degree to completing residency,[37] and Jacob Simpson, as well as the modern-day counterparts of the "boys in white," frequently achieve this. When I asked Simpson, a thirty-five-year-old internal medicine and infectious diseases expert, how he became a doctor, he replied, "I didn't experience the challenges that other Latino physicians might have. . . . I don't fit the traditional narrative." Jacob, who self-identified as Hispanic and was wearing a small Colombia flag pin on one of the flaps of his white coat, was curious about how I found him. "I have a white name, and I look like a white male. Did you find me through a physician call bank or some other mechanism?" It had been a referral from someone who knew him.[38]

Jacob's appearance and Anglo-sounding name were not the only characteristics that made him stand out among the Latina/o doctors. Most were first-generation college students from working-class origins whose parents worked as housekeepers, plumbers, gardeners, or factory workers. Jacob was born in Armenia, Colombia, but had no recollection or any information about his biological parents. Records of his parents most likely burned when the Palacio de Justicia was torched in 1985 by guerrilla fighters.[39] A foster family in Bogotá that owned a small business took care of him until he was about a year old, when an affluent Jewish American family who lived in Missouri adopted him, conferring US citizenship on him. He was raised in Missouri and attended K-12 schools there. Jacob's birth name was José María Paz, but his adoptive parents, a clinical social worker, and a cardiologist, changed it to "a more Caucasian sounding name" during the adoption process. With no access to Spanish/English bilingual education programs in his K-12 schooling, he double majored in Spanish literature/ Latin American history and biochemistry at Arizona State University, with a deep desire to reconnect and reestablish some of his heritage even as he pursued medicine. For his residency training, he opted to attend schools in regions like Texas and Florida, places where he felt he would come across more Latinos. His parents, who were highly educated professionals, helped pay his way, but he also took out loans. He was one of the few doctors I interviewed who was a certified bilingual doctor by dint of having taken an exam[40] to establish his fluency.

Beyond his parents' financial support, Jacob benefited from his father's cultural and social capital. He was the sole USMG in my sample who had a physician parent educated and trained in America.[41] Jacob's adoptive father was an interventional cardiologist who had run his private practice for over thirty years. Jacob visited his father's office frequently throughout his youth and he saw his father "navigate his own medical hurdles" as the sole owner and practitioner. In some ways, Jacob's higher education narrative parallels those of the white men medical students described in *Boys in White*. Medical students at the University of Kansas in the early 1960s, the "boys in white" consisted primarily of young men from middle-class homes with college-educated fathers, and nearly 20 percent were the sons of a doctor.[42] However, Jacob's experience contrasted with Latin American IMGs who migrated to the US as highly skilled professionals. Below, I highlight the narratives of a few Latin American IMGs who were offered (and/or sought) an opportunity in US medicine and then began the process of taking the licensing exam[43] to legally work in the United States with a high-skill visa that some American universities and hospitals provided.

## POSITIVELY SELECTED LATIN AMERICAN IMGS

Positively selected Latin American IMGs were able to bypass some of the institutional barriers that Latina/o USMGs encountered. While physicians or STEM professionals trained in Latin America have a harder time translating degrees and recertifying themselves—a process called nativist credentialism—some are positively selected and opt to "re-do" medical school.[44] Mateo's father, a Peruvian-trained urologist and IMG, did this when he migrated in 1963. Mateo, now also a urologist but a USMG, followed in his father's footsteps and benefited from working alongside his father over the summer by developing X-rays or helping him review charts. Mateo revealed that he got angry when he learned that his father had to complete "extra work" to practice in America. For his part, his father was glad not to be working at the gas station where he started upon arrival before beginning a medical residency in the US. Their perspectives about the situation contrasted significantly.

Positively selected immigrants are those who are highly educated in their countries of origin and can secure highly skilled (H-1B or J-1) visas to work or study in America.[45] The J-1 visa, I came to learn, was referred to as *"la jota de jodido"* [akin to the f of fucked] in Marisol's networks. While some physicians trained in other countries experience downward mobility and work as taxi drivers in New York or makeshift offices in their homes and garages,[46] Marisol applied for a J visa upon gaining a fellowship to further her training at Harvard Medical School once she finished her schooling in Colombia. To waive the two-year requirement, she applied for an exceptionally skilled visa and requested letters from Harvard and her home country's educational institution to demonstrate her unparalleled human capital skills. Marisol explained that she paid more to the immigration lawyer ($10,000) who helped her with her case than when obtaining her medical schooling in Colombia, which was free for her as the daughter of an educator.

Immigrants are selected along multiple lines such as for their high educational levels, like South Asian doctors in England,[47] or for their labor in low-wage sectors, like Mexican immigrant men who worked as part of the Bracero Program.[48] Because of the high level of education they had attained before pre-migration, IMGs were "positively selected" by US institutions. Among the eleven international medical graduate doctors in the sample, only one did not have professional and highly educated parents; his parents worked in a small store and as a mechanic. The rest were part of the professional or middle class. Foreign-born women IMGs initially sought programs in the United States because they wanted "more" advancement and were then offered opportunities by employers and institutions that wanted to keep, retain, and invest in them.

Marisol sought this advancement in her specialty. Elsa, a gastroenterologist, also arrived in the US in her early thirties because she wanted to advance in her career. She told me that she had already finished medical training and completed a specialization in Colombia but came to the US because she "wanted to do research." She found a physician in Canada and sent him an email about joining his lab. He invited her to join, and she worked in Canada for a year and a half. Elsa was highly sought after for her skills and a university in Colombia offered her an assistant professor position to teach medicine and gastroenterology, so she went home for three more years. She then returned to Canada but found a cooperative research effort between a university in Canada and a facility in Cleveland, Ohio. Recognizing that she was "the only person" other than an engineer who knew how to manage a machine that was an artificial pacemaker to make the bowels and the stomach move, she transferred to a clinic in Cleveland. She explained, "I wanted to be independent. I wanted to be the principal investigator [of my research projects]. I wanted to be able to determine what I want to do when I want to do it, and I decided to repeat my training." This meant that Elsa had to take the USMLE test. Once she passed, she matched in Seattle in internal medicine for residency and then a top university for gastroenterology.

Sociologist Tanya Jenkins has found that non-USMDs must significantly outperform American medical degree counterparts to gain admission to residency programs and often end up in training programs of lesser prestige. She suggests that all IMGs nonetheless continue to experience disadvantages.[49] The few Latina/o IMGs I interviewed, most of them women, offered competing accounts of how their social class pre-migration, as well as their phenotype (a point I discuss in chapter 6), influenced their outlooks. "I guess they saw potential and hired me after I finished," Elsa said. She reflected, "I don't know how inspirational it's going to be for young people living here but at least it's another way to come to this system." IMGs are not a homogenous group,[50] but Elsa acknowledged that Latina/o USMGs had difficulty gaining access to the wealth of opportunities she gained.

In Latin America, students who enter medical school do so right after high school, which significantly lowers the cost and the time to degree. "We do not have college. . . . I finished high school and went directly to medicine," Maria a Peruvian IMG, explained. The median time to degree for doctors who received their medical degrees in Latin America was seven years, with the sixth year being the intern year and the seventh the social service year. Moreover, the cost of their schooling is between $7,000-$10,000 US in total. Cynthia noted the affordability in Perú: "We paid per semester, per each unit. . . . It did not exceed 500 soles. How much would it be in dollars? It was so little. I studied in a public university, not a private one." In 2021, 500 soles would amount to $126.00 every semester. This low cost of university schooling allowed Cynthia to focus on her studies and not have to work. Her parents financially supported her via their successful small business until she finished establishing her career. Additionally, Armando, in internal medicine, attended public medical school in Mexico and was working as a doctor in Long Beach, CA at the time of the interview. He said, "It was about 1,000 pesos ($58.65) per semester." For comparison, the average approximate cost of attending medical school in France is 450 euros (roughly $500) per year, and in Germany up to 3500 euros ($3800) yearly.

US medicine considers any doctor an IMG if they studied abroad, even if they are US citizens. This is exemplified by Gabriel, who was born in Chula Vista, CA, a city along the San Diego/Tijuana border, and who had a transborder student experience. While Gabriel completed kinder-garten to ninth grade in the US, he finished high school across the border in Tijuana, Mexico at an American-affiliated private school called CETYS (*Centro de Enseñanza Ténica y Superior*). Gabriel's father, a businessman, paid for all of his schooling in Mexico, including his tuition at the Auton-omous University of Baja California, which was $500.00 every year for seven years of medical training. A departure from working-class Latina/o USMGs, Gabriel wasn't expected to be the financial safety net for this family. "I was not working, I had no rent, and no loans to pay." In the end, he moved to Massachusetts to complete his medical residency.

When I asked Jazmín how she came to practice in the United States, she said that it started when she applied for a prestigious postdoctoral fellowship to work with a leading figure in dermatology. She was fifty-one at the time of the interview and had been in the United States since she was thirty. She had gone to medical school and done her residency at the Universidad Pontificia Bolivariana, a private university in Colom-bia. Her mother was a practicing physician there and her father worked as an accountant. One of her siblings was also a doctor in Colombia. When her research fellowship was nearing the end, she was offered a tenure-track clinical professor position at a top-ranking University of California institution, contingent on her passing the USMLE, which as Jazmín had noted was very "tough" for her because "it was a lot of working, a lot of studying" to do in a short timeframe of six months. She did. Jazmín felt very fortunate because she knew it was "a great opportunity" for her, she told me a couple of times.[51]

The same opportunity was presented to Isabel, an IMG who trained at *Universidade Federal de Minas Gerais* in Brazil via a fellowship.[52] She was trilingual and self-identified as Latina.[53] Isabel received training in radiology in Boston for one year and then returned to Brazil and practiced there for three years. She was thirty when she returned to the United States because her employer in Boston created an avenue for her to practice in California, which was to do a fellowship in pediatric radiology. This gave her the opportunity to start the "complicated" process of getting her medical school degree "validated" and her license to practice in California, necessary to enter a tenure-track job. Isabel took all the exams and then was able to stay on as faculty at a major research university.

Unlike the rest of the highly educated Latin American women physicians who were looking to move, Cynthia said that she had never contemplated it. Her husband, however, a practicing lawyer and theologian in Perú, was invited to teach at a religious school in Los Angeles. The whole family was then invited to come along with him as he preached. Cynthia noted that the transition "was easy. [My husband] came as a resident and then we all were residents because we came as a married couple with three children. We got residency [status] quickly due to that situation." Cynthia was in her late forties when the family moved to La Puente, California, in 1989, and knew that she would not be able to practice medicine in the United States unless she prepared and recertified herself. Cynthia contacted the Education Commission for Foreign Medical Graduates in Perú and they gave her the steps to follow and how to prepare to practice medicine in the US.

The narratives of positively selected IMGs trained in Latin America reflect how institutions of higher education, especially in medicine, have career outlets built in that they were able to pursue as highly skilled immigrants. But rather than the institutions merely opening up to them by providing them with a job, the context of their medical education in Perú, Colombia, Mexico, or Brazil had been vastly different. Most were professional or middle class, but perhaps most importantly, they did not have to contend with racial discrimination and legal status precarity or with having had subpar K-9 schooling. These advancement opportunities were not as readily available to most Latina/o USMGs who had received most or all their schooling and training in America, who experienced circuitous paths into the field, and who had amassed an absurd amount of debt which they were expected to pay off by attaining a high salaried career.

Socioeconomic status produces circuitous paths into the profession for USMG Latina/o doctors and straight-line paths for positively selected Latin American IMGs who show evidence of unparalleled high skills. Unlike Becker's white male medical students who went "straight from college into medical school,"[54] Latina/o USMG physicians' paths' were interrupted by institutionalized discrimination in K-12 schooling and the strains of their socioeconomic class position in their immigrant families. Their paths were circuitous and marked by significant delays, as they had to scrounge up solutions each time a new structural blockade in the pipeline presented itself. They also amassed a significant amount of debt that forced them to take lengthy pauses throughout their training as familial financial urgencies remained. On the other hand, a few elite Latina/o international medical graduate students and physicians who met all requirements were able to enter American medicine in what Latina/o USMGs perceived to be a more direct fashion, via opportunities embedded into institutions of higher education in the US that are not readily accessible to the poorer and minoritized physicians who are educated in American schools. To be sure, Latin American IMGs experienced costly immigration roadblocks, but in ways different than Marisa, whose initial undocumented status produced a significant weight and strain that added more time and financial hardship to her journey and produced cumulative disadvantages for her that spilled over to her family.

Data sources like the AMA Physician Masterfile data, which do not include intra-ethnic measures of race and ethnicity, cannot wholly capture the cultural and structural racism that all Latina/o doctors, regardless of nativity, face en route to American medicine. Institutions of higher education must disaggregate the first-generation college student experience to develop adequate supports. A qualitative intra-Latina/o dynamics lens reveals that while both first-generation college-educated men and women faced similar circuitous paths, they contrast heavily with positively selected Latin American physicians who received their graduate medical training in other countries. Positively selected Latin American IMGs were able to bypass the economic hardships and institutionalized racism that those attending US schools had to navigate. Here, we can see the polyvalence of the white coat operating for both USMG and IMG Latina/o doctors, who often get subsumed under the same pan-ethnic category. Foreign-trained Latina/o physicians who were positively selected by research universities or large hospitals were able to enter the occupation because colleges and universities that needed their exceptional expertise granted or created opportunities for them. While other scholars note that IMGs may be perceived as less qualified by patients and coworkers,[55] here we see that Latina/o USMGs perceived Latin American IMGs to be held in higher regard than they were. This sentiment is fueled by the lackluster efforts to provide systemic supports for underrepresented people of color in STEM in the US and how they are racialized in the American and educational systems.

In the next chapter, I give the reader an insider view of how social capital networks became more consequential for Latina/o physicians as they moved up the higher echelons of the US educational hierarchy and through medical school. The active maintenance of structural barriers by various social actors exemplifies how finding just one significant mentor or pan-ethnic organization could be critical for aspiring Latina/o physicians, considering the anemic efforts by institutions to address them. I offer their perspectives on the hoops they had to jump through in this system to locate *one* mentor or program in the higher education pipeline that would take the time and make the effort to guide them through the entire process. These networks were gendered and racialized and relied heavily on linguistic capital.

# 4.

# GENDERED NETWORKS AND LINGUISTIC CAPITAL

> Mentorship was vital in my path to medicine. My family and friends broke their backs to afford me the chance to study for twelve years and defer income. My mentors supported me and opened doors, pushed back ideas of persistent impostor syndrome, and buffered the roller coaster ride. My family was the engine/car, my mentors were the GPS. You can't go nowhere [*sic*] without both pieces.
>
> —ALEJANDRO CRUZ, Internal Medicine

THE INTERVIEWS SHOW that the key point of intervention for Latina/o physicians to counteract the effects of institutionalized racism in higher education is the influence of at least "one truly significant other"[1] in American colleges and universities. These truly significant others—either individuals or ethnic-based organizations—shared the "game book" with respondents at a time when structural obstacles and social actors weighed aspiring Latina/o doctors down or held them back by actively maintaining and upholding structural barriers that favored white masculinist norms and metrics in medicine. Latina/o physicians and medical graduate students—who were taking courses, rotations, and selecting specialties—indicated that finding just one mentor or ethnic-based medical program in higher education that invested a significant amount of time in them was pivotal to their advancement in health-related arenas. In the face of institutionalized racism, both men and women turned to their ethnic and cultural strengths to navigate the structures that contributed to their marginalization; however, women were more able to leverage their gendered linguistic capital to gain opportunities and develop health-related networks at this stage than were men who experienced disadvantage.

These dynamics are exemplified by Alejandro, the US-born son of Mexican immigrants, and now an internal medicine doctor. "If you don't have connections to medicine good fucking luck getting meaningful shadowing experiences," he said to me. He was frustrated, and he dropped several F-bombs during the interview, describing the difficulties he and other first-generation college Latinas/os encounter. He described interactions with a volunteer coordinator at the hospital in his hometown who initially relegated him to being a greeter, cleaning gurneys, or walking elderly patients to their cars instead of shadowing doctor-patient interactions. Alejandro retorted, "Look, I'm not gonna drive here for two hours to walk old people to their cars." A series of uncomfortable interactions ensued as she recommended other unskilled positions that were available. Alejandro recalled that with a buzz cut and a thick black mustache at the time, he was likely stereotyped as poor and uneducated. He described the volunteer coordinator saying, "Well I thought that you were from Salinas?" referencing an agricultural city that's the backdrop of John Steinbeck's The Grapes of Wrath. When he said he was from Salinas but didn't live there and that he lived in Berkeley, she seemed confused. "Berkeley? What are you doing there?" Alejandro retorted, "I go to college there. I go to UC Berkeley."

> She looks at me with a *pinche cara de pendejo* [fuckin' dumbass face]. 'Oh, you do? That's fantastic! Did I tell you that I have a niece that goes there?' Blah, blah, blah. Don't try to connect with me now, *ya te chingastes* [you fucked yourself]! That opportunity is gone. Then she gives me a shirt and

says 'Here you go. Here's your name tag.' She walked me to the ER, around the ER, giving me a little tour.

Alejandro's difficulties continued in the ER. "I might as well have been a fly on the wall. *Nadien me pelaba.* [No one acknowledged me]." Nonetheless, "I would go on Friday, Friday night, Saturday, and Sunday. Then I would drive back to undergrad at Berkeley." Each visit involved two hours of driving each way. But despite this diligence, Alejandro did not become visible to the doctors empowered to give him access to meaningful training experiences until he spoke up when a doctor was flipping channels between sports games, and he asked the doctor, who was white, to return to Berkeley's football game. Alejandro recalled,

He looked at me like 'Who the fuck is talking to me?' He said, 'Why?' I said, 'Because the Cal game is on. What do you care? That's my team.' He said, 'Which one?' 'Cal!' I said. And he was like, 'Why is that your team?' And I said, 'cuz I go there.' And he's like, 'Go where?' I responded, 'I go to Berkeley.' And you know, he's still looking at me like *cara de pendejo* [dumbass face]. 'I am a student at UC Berkeley. That is my team. Go Bears!' He goes, 'Oh, you go to Cal?' And I responded, 'Yeah.' And he's like 'Huh?!' 'I'm here as a volunteer. I'm from Salinas. And I'm here to get experience,' I replied. 'Oh, you're not here as part of the county program?' the doctor said. . . . 'Oh, well I'm from the Bay. Come with me. You want to see this.'

Alejandro explained the county program to me:

A judge would send the youth to a wing in the hospital that housed drug abuse patients as part of a court-ordered county program. There were kids my age-ish . . . that were there because they were caught with drug offenses. The judge would send you to the emergency room as part of your probation so that you can see people come in on overdoses. Better than jail time. He [the doctor] and I don't know how many others thought that I was there on a court order as opposed to me being a volunteer. Even though my shirt said, volunteer.

It was evident that employees at the hospital did not think Alejandro fit into the traditional medical student archetype—white, male, and middle class. They presumed he was not a pre-medical student until he mentioned Cal Berkeley, one of the most prestigious institutions in the country, and then they peppered him with questions before they could locate him within their understanding of prospective doctors. Alejandro endured these racialized slights and continued to receive mentorship from the ER doctor because he desperately needed and wanted the experience. These racialized harms and slights were an added weight that he had to bear, and he found some relief when he came across a program at Berkeley aimed at diversifying underrepresented groups in STEM. Now that he is a doctor himself, Alejandro had created a pan-ethnic mentorship and shadowing program at the hospital where he was employed to provide aspiring pre-health Latine students a roadmap into medicine and what he described as "meaningful shadowing experiences." He now served as an empowerment agent—a mentor who possessed the relevant experiential knowledge, critical consciousness, and navigational capital—and had developed an important hub that could help budding doctors build their social capital.[2] Most men doctors that were either 1.5 or second generation, whether they were older or more recent graduates, had experiences like Alejandro.[3]

In many ways, Vilna Bashi's hubs-and-spokes metaphor for West Indian immigrant networks and their connections to social mobility and jobs is useful here.[4] In Bashi's model, immigrant veterans in places such as New York, London, and the West Indies are the hubs in search of immigrant newcomers (the spokes) to recommend for jobs and other opportunities. I focus on the inverse; in my model, Latina/o physicians are the spokes in search of a network hub.

I argue that social capital networks become more consequential as aspiring Latina/o physicians move up the higher rungs of the educational hierarchy and through medical school into specialties. I focus on the obstacles they faced finding mentors, the network hubs that could leverage their weight, connections, and reputations to find aspiring Latinas/os positions in medical fields that otherwise would not exist for many of those who were the first in their families to attend college. The different forms of support from mentors and ethnic-based programs influenced how Latina/o clinicians experienced training and were placed, blocked, or steered into opportunities that networked them into primary care (family, internal, or pediatric medicine) by faculty, mentors, and graduate ethnic medical programs. This situation has created an occupational sorting influenced by the intersection of their ethnic linguistic capital strengths and gender.

## FINDING HUBS: ENCOUNTERING GATEKEEPING, INSTITUTIONAL, OR EMPOWERMENT AGENTS

In navigating the circuitous pathways toward medical school, as I showed in the previous chapter, finding one mentor or program that was firmly embedded in the medical ecosystem or knew the inner workings of the field was the anchor that physicians explained could harness their support to provide them with access to their networks.[5] Latinas/os that were the first in their family to pursue health careers could rarely find that support in their families of origin. "I think some parents [can] say 'Oh that's great! Why don't I call my friend who's already a doctor and ask him to help you,'" indicated Paolo, currently an internal medicine doctor who was raised by Mexican immigrant parents who worked in a dry cleaning plant, to highlight his lack of ties to high-status mentors and networks compared to some of his former classmates. Built-in institutionalized discrimination also resulted in a dearth of co-ethnic STEM faculty mentors that they could rely on as well.

We know that support is vital to social mobility and that a lack of high-social-capital networks can reproduce social inequality. Institutions or individual agents, such as professors or networks embedded within organizations in colleges, can intercede and open pathways that were previously nebulous to students.[6] Education sociologist Ricardo Stanton-Sálazar identifies three types of social agents that disrupt or sustain the inequality created by disparities in social capital.[7] These include gatekeeping, institutional, and empowerment agents. Gatekeeping agents are high-status individuals who determine access to the halls of power. They maintain the status quo by supporting the aspirations of people who strongly align with or exhibit the characteristics that are valued by a white mainstream dominant culture. They contrast with institutional agents, who are non-familial individuals who use their high-status positions, capital, or personal networks to provide low-status students with institutional support that helps them reach the higher echelons of the educational hierarchy. Institutional support can be understood as resources and social support that allow individuals to effectively navigate institutional systems and expand the opportunities available to them. Empowerment agents fulfill the same roles as institutional agents, but they propagate a social justice agenda and possess a critical consciousness. Mentors with a critical consciousness understand the many ways social, political, and economic forms of oppression limit life chances and challenge them. Stanton-Sálazar contends that empowerment agents are any institutional agent with a critical consciousness. However, empowerment agent roles are fulfilled differently based on social location because marginalized students interpret and connect to the particular experiential knowledge (based on shared commonalities of race/ethnicity, class, and gender) these agents offer in different ways.

## "You Don't Fit the Profile!": Encountering Gatekeeping Agents

Latina/o physicians recalled experiences with individuals of various racial/ethnic backgrounds who acted as gatekeepers as they sought entry and moved through medical school, such as the volunteer coordinator and the white physician Alejandro described. These gatekeepers dissuaded or discouraged them from pursuing valuable opportunities that would propel them forward. Gatekeeping agents usually limit their support because of racialized, gendered, and classed biases. Institutional agents can become gatekeeping agents by stereotyping Latine students as less academically competent despite providing important institutional support. For Latinas/os pursuing medicine, these gatekeeping agents were not limited to one particular social category—they were of various backgrounds and highlighted how Latine and non-Latines engage in upholding culturally biased metrics that are often valued by the US medical system and hegemonic ideas of Latines in science.

Some gatekeepers were co-ethnics, which disheartened aspiring physicians. Marisa, the Central American pathologist introduced in the previous chapter, learned that she had to network to gain access to medical opportunities, and only along the way did she realize that she had none while some of her peers had ample resources to draw from.

> I would have to do that uncomfortable thing of networking. That is my weakness. I'm always afraid that I don't deserve that extra help from someone. I've had to accomplish things on my own. At this level networking is key. It's who you know. I never knew that I didn't [know] anybody. . . . I've always had to ask for letters of recommendation from my professors because I didn't have anybody outside of that. . . . These other kids [are] like, 'I'll ask my dad's colleague in their office to write me a letter.'

Aware of the popular dictum "It's not what you know, but who you know," she scheduled a meeting with a Latine dean of diversity at an Ivy League university to seek support in an attempt to expand her network. She recalled:

> I told [the dean] my story. I told him my [MCAT] score, and he was like, 'Well, even if you took it again, most people don't raise their score more than three or four points at the most. Maybe you should start looking into nursing or something else.' Like, make a separate plan. That was so

disheartening. It hit me hard. I drove all the way from [the university] to my . . . house crying. But then it pissed me off. . . . I was like, 'No! I've been pursuing this. I know I can do it.' And then [that private Ivy] was no longer my dream school. I brought my score up by ten points. It's almost like I did it to show him.

Anger motivated Marisa. Eventually, she gained admission to a prominent public school where she was the sole Latina in her program, but it took a significant amount of time for her to regroup and regain her confidence before doing so. As her experience demonstrates, even co-ethnic gatekeepers can possess culturally deficient perspectives, such as blaming educational disparities on students' families or cultures, while failing to acknowledge the role of structural discrimination in institutions or of culturally biased tests that are ill-suited to predict eventual success.[8]

Many gatekeepers are affiliated with US institutions, and the physicians in the sample who completed their schooling in the United States told me it was common to be shunned by potential mentors, or to be continually discouraged or turned away by people who they hoped would help them. The older cohort of physicians that attended institutions of higher education just past the 1970s was more likely to narrate explicit forms of exclusion—racial and gender discrimination—while more recent physicians noted it was subtle. These younger doctors also sought or had access to ethnic-affirming spaces. Cecilia, a successful cardiologist who pursued medical school in the 1980s, was told that she "could never be a doctor because she was too dumb and Hispanic" from various people. Yalitza, who was Honduran and Salvadoran and had more recently graduated with degrees in social welfare and education, recounted how various gatekeeping agents reacted negatively to her plans to pursue medicine through a postbaccalaureate program designed to make students more competitive:

I did an internship, and it was public health based. We would have to work with one of the physicians there [and] talk to her about our career goals. I told her, 'I want to do a postbacc.' She asked, 'What is your GPA?' I told her. She said, 'That's not high enough. Don't you know how competitive they are? The percentage [of schools] that you'll get into?' That kind of brought down my hopes for trying to go to medical school.

Yalitza followed through anyway because other people not in medicine supported her. The response from college counselors and the physician at the internship she interacted with was typical among individuals in STEM programs in that they often use grade point averages and exam scores to evaluate academic performance and success in these fields, despite research showing these measures are racially and ethnically biased and do not determine program completion.[9] Whenever she would ask for guidance, Janet felt that she received more discouragement than encouragement, and various people would point her to different careers. While friends and family were crucial to overcoming these setbacks, they lacked the kind of capital that opened doors into the profession. Janet summarized this succinctly when she said that her pathway into medicine "wasn't very guided."

After they earned admission into US medical schools, many of the Latinas/os in my sample indicated that they were monitored by high-status gatekeepers who felt they should not be there. Ivan, now in emergency medicine, appreciated that the sole medical school he applied to, and ultimately enrolled in, used a holistic approach in their selection process.[10] The admissions committee took into consideration the significant health-care-based work he had already undertaken with minority communities. When he began the program, however, the dean of admissions called him in to speak with her about what she saw as his inadequate MCAT scores. Ivan is soft-spoken; he had none of Alejandro's bluster. As he recounted, the dean told him, "'You don't fit the profile.' She told me that 'I didn't deserve to be there and that I was taking someone's spot'" Ivan recounted. The dean said that she was going to "keep a close eye on him" and that any little shift she saw in his performance would be grounds for program dismissal. Ivan, the son of Mexican-heritage parents, took this to mean that he "got in through a back door that was well guarded." This scrutiny made him doubt his capabilities as he felt that he was filling a race-based quota, even though he was admitted in 2014 to a program specifically designed to train physicians who wanted to work with underserved Latine communities. He struggled to feel like he belonged in medicine for several years. When we spoke, Ivan, who was in medical school a decade ago and was now one of the few in his specialty in Fresno, California, said that he sometimes suffered from impostor syndrome—the feelings of personal incompetence that persist despite clear evidence of competence.

Armando, in internal medicine, also internalized the discouragement of a gatekeeper. As an IMG who was trained at a public university in Mexico on a scholarship, Armando felt that he carried a "stigma of being a foreign graduate and not being competitive enough." Because he grew up poor in a city in Mexico with parents who were raised in a small rural village, Armando felt he was heavily stigmatized in America. He was also a gay Mexican man. Armando had no plans to emigrate to the United States until he met his future husband during the last year of medical school and the couple had to decide who would move. Armando ended up in the US in 2010 and began the recertification process, such as taking the USMLE test. He was advised not to give any indication that he was gay in his medical school applications. Armando had to reapply for a visa three times, and he only succeeded when his employer, a large HMO in Northern California, sponsored him for legal permanent residency.[11] He envisioned applying to a range of medical schools and aiming for top-tier places to complete the fellowship that could negate all stigma.[12] Tanya M. Jenkins notes that status hierarchies are developed further in medicine based on where students received their medical degree. She argues that those who were considered international medical graduates push USMGs higher in the hierarchy and into elite training positions.[13] Armando's program director encouraged him to seek the advice of the chief of medicine about applying to Ivy League schools, as she had attended one. Her response to his plan shocked him:

> The chief of medicine said, 'You shouldn't do that. You should adjust your applications based on whatever you think you might fit.' She was saying to aim for smaller hospitals . . . hospitals that historically have taken people from other countries. . . . That was shocking to me. It was disheartening. She was in the field that I wanted to go into. . . . I felt like she was right. I'm like, 'Oh my God! What am I doing? Maybe I should go for something that's going to be more for sure? To be more realistic?'

Armando went home and reflected on her words. "I thought about it again. I'm like, 'Wait a minute!' This is like the biggest mental barrier that someone is putting on you," and it made him irate. Ultimately, Armando did not heed her advice and applied broadly. He ended up doing an elective at one of the Harvard-affiliated hospitals for three months, and then he was accepted for another prestigious fellowship at Brown University. "I was very mad at [the chief of medicine who had discouraged him] afterward because it's not fair. . . . You can't be a mentor when you are limiting your mentees' goals, expectations, dreams." He indicated the significance of such failures when he said, "I think that is, by far, one of the worst examples I can give of discrimination in a way." While Armando was aware that he "started at the top" in comparison to other poor and immigrant Latinos in terms of his social mobility, he felt that the medical world saw him through a different lens, as his foreign medical credentials, class upbringing, and sexual orientation influenced how other medical professionals saw him. Indeed, for respondents, fighting off demoralizing guidance and racial injury from crucial gatekeepers had taken time and a toll on their progress.

## Really Significant Others: Institutional and Empowerment Agents

Because first-generation Latina/o college students had difficulties developing high-social-capital networks in their families of origin and bumped across gatekeeping agents repeatedly, they relied on a few, select, institutional agents—high-status, often non-kin individuals who occupy relatively powerful institutional positions, and who are well positioned to provide key forms of social and institutional support—to procure access to educational and workplace opportunities. The French sociologist Pierre Bourdieu theorized that all forms of capital are related. Social capital (such as relationships with teachers, peers, or family members) can be used to access economic or cultural capital. That is resources like advice, institutional knowledge, or academic skills, which can then be harnessed to generate human capital (such as educational success and credentials). While virtually all individuals possess some form of social capital, it is socially stratified along multiple dimensions,[14] with those from working-class origins having less bridging capital than their privileged counterparts, as bridging capital offers greater access to diverse and valued information that facilitates social mobility. This is especially true for Latine college students pursuing STEM, since there is an alarming dearth of Latina/o professional mentors available to them.[15]

Olga, a proud member of the National Hispanic Medical Association, described the lack of co-ethnic mentors thus:

Most medical students make it because they have support within the medical school to keep going. Even if they have problems with individuals, if they hit roadblocks, or can't pass exams. . . . [T]here's so many roadblocks, but you can still pick yourself up and keep going with the support of others around you—the faculty, the Minority Affairs office staff, Latino and older students. But [Latines are] not leading. We're not deans in medical schools. We're not on the boards at hospitals. We're not in leadership positions.

Yet, established mentors of any background can provide aspiring medical doctors with networks and instrumental support to help them get their foot in the door once they have successfully navigated the circuitous and lengthy pathways into medical school. Chicana feminist scholar Aida Hurtado found that Chicanas in science benefited from a collective web of support from parents, extended family, and community members. Their testimonios revealed that success was enhanced by relationship-centered, validating actions of teachers and mentors who provided encouragement, guidance, and affirmation.[16] But for Latinos/as pursuing medicine, these institutional agents were scarce, so their mentors were often non-Latines in science, or Latinas/os in other fields of study. In some cases, initial gatekeeping agents who attempted to block Latinas/os from opportunities turned into institutional agents.

### "Someone Gave Me a Chance": Men and Social Networks

Institutional agents provided important behind-the-scenes information and access to a hidden curriculum in medicine. Samuel, the US-born child of Peruvian immigrants, acknowledged this. I interviewed Samuel in between his check-ins with patients. Samuel told me that his immigrant parents[17] first settled in the Mission District in San Francisco, California, but that the family decided to move to East Bay in Walnut Creek, which was a more affluent area and where most residents were either Asian or white. This plan did not produce what they intended—promoting upward social mobility—as Samuel found himself on a downwardly mobile path[18] and was spending time with young people who were doing "bad stuff" in the "streets." It was "the wrong crowd," he said. He graduated from high school with a GPA in the 2.0 range but excelled at Diablo Community College which he attended for two years, earning a 3.9 grade point average. "I timed it well," he said, in that he was intentional about the classes he selected and was able to get all of his requirements done within a two-year time frame to transfer into UC Berkeley's Molecular Cell Biology program. But when he graduated from Cal an academic mentor told him that a 3.1 GPA in his major was "not good enough to get into any California medical school," and he did not apply. Samuel reasoned he "needed more time" and "more experience." He sought a job but was unable to find steady white-collar employment after college and he worked a series of odd jobs such as making sandwiches at Togo's and also picking up dog poop at a kennel. He also taught sex education classes at the Boys and Girls Club, ran a mentorship program that brought students from Berkeley to underserved areas in the Mission District, and obtained an opportunity in a lab at a major research university in San Francisco curating mice for a genetics study. Still interested in attending medical school, Samuel applied for a paid shadowing position at San Francisco General Hospital but was limited to "handing out juices and blankets to patients."

Over time, Samuel came across a South Asian Indian plastic surgeon who became his "first real mentor" through the shadowing position. He described it as a serendipitous fluke of fate, but the connection was bound to happen as a paid employee in a hospital. This really significant other invested in Samuel, reading his medical school application and giving him feedback. When Samuel applied to do his surgical residency at a private highly selective university, he was rejected. This mentor told him that he could appeal the decision and guided him through the entire process of writing and submitting the appeal letter. His mentor also wrote a formal letter to the admissions committee as well, and the decision was reversed. Samuel recognized that his mentor's letter had "carrie[d] a lot of weight." It was this empowerment agent and physician who taught Samuel the hidden curriculum of higher education.

Because the demands of their jobs are onerous, doctors who serve as hubs have to be selective and can only mentor one or a few people at a given point in time.[19] According to respondents, shadowing at a health-care facility is a prime way of making connections in medicine and getting doors open. Julio observed that some of his white and East Asian peers were able to find meaningful shadowing experiences by relying on relatives to provide them. Homogeneous peer networks may function well for capital-rich groups such as upper-middle-class whites and East Asian immigrants, but they are less helpful for under-resourced groups like working-class individuals, Blacks, and Latinas/os.[20] Resources readily available to students whose parents are in the sciences and/or well-off financially are critical to internships and summer jobs that can change a student's life trajectory and ultimate success in STEM.[21] The "hubs" guide the "spokes" to and through medical programs. Hubs can provide access to behind-the-scenes information, arrange employment opportunities, and continuously help students with a range of needs.

Ivan, who still struggled with impostor syndrome, found himself working at Bed, Bath and Beyond after earning a Bachelor of Science in biology with a 2.5 GPA. However, he maintained connections to his undergraduate university by applying to be a volunteer for medical research programs. He accessed a valuable network when he was hired to join the lab of a white cardiothoracic surgeon. In this lab, he met an African American man who promised to mentor him if he could bring his MCAT scores up. This mentor held only a high school diploma and initially worked as a janitor in the facility, but the cardiothoracic surgeon who oversaw the lab had noticed his dexterity with his hands and hired him to do skilled work. Ivan learned how to do heart transplants on rabbits from this individual. Ivan related, "He taught me how to [suture], anesthesia, and ventilation on different animal models. Everything applicable in the clinical setting." Ivan credited this mentor for sharing meaningful clinical training exercises that made it possible for him to become a stronger candidate come application season.

Benito's mentor was more along the line of Samuel's. "Someone gave me a chance," he gratefully told me. That "someone" was Dr. Noé

Sandoval,[22] an associate clinical professor in family medicine in the University of California system who was of Mexican heritage. This co-ethnic physician took Benito under his wing and helped him navigate school and seek out opportunities. Dr. Sandoval expended various resources and time and pulled strings for Benito. Perhaps not incidentally for an empowerment agent, Dr. Sandoval's research was on factors that impact career selection in the health professions among minority students. For starters, he placed Benito in a STEM-focused dormitory. All residents of the dorm took a class designed to help first-generation college students acclimate to campus life, but in Benito's class, only about a quarter of enrollees completed college. Benito felt like a "lone survivor." Dr. Sandoval connected him to family health clinics in lower-income communities with large Latine populations where he could shadow, an experience Benito found inspiring and meaningful.

Dr. Sandoval died when Benito was off completing his residency requirements but before that, Benito described his difficulties gaining meaningful shadowing experiences without the help of a mentor. Meaningful shadowing experiences or conducting clinical research are a crucial part of the hidden curriculum for gaining entry to medical schools.[23] Much like Alejandro, he was initially assigned menial work. However, when he connected with Dr. Sandoval, who was of Mexican origin, bilingual, and who had worked to support his studies at local grocery stores by packing grapes each summer in Delano, CA, he stumbled across an empowerment agent. When we spoke, Benito had gained an opportunity to work in the same building and clinic where Dr. Sandoval worked, and his gratitude was boundless. "The exact clinic where I [shadowed my mentor] is the exact building I'm sitting in today and overseeing," he said.

Thus far the examples in this chapter have been of men, a few of whom worked as interpreters to gain entry and experience, but in the sample, this was a common occurrence among women.

## Gendered Networks: Women and Linguistic Capital

Women were more likely to attain volunteer or paid positions in small clinics, hospitals, or educational institutions as interpreters, a key way to build networks. Some worked as medical scribes. Ana explained that she took advantage of a work opportunity to be a translator for medical residents.

> I became a translator for UCI medical residents. . . . The residents would see the patient and I would be in the middle translating back and forth between the patient and the physician. I thought to myself, 'Gosh, I speak Spanish. I could be directly speaking to the patient while they are being seen or treated.'

Unlike men, who were initially relegated to cleaning duties in their shadowing positions, women could leverage their gender identities and linguistic capital to obtain health-related experiences in ways that men struggled to do. This bilingual linguistic capital has been shown to benefit biliterate women who may gain valuable skills that are rewarded in school and the labor market.[24] For example, when Rosalva, a Peruvian first-generation college student, enrolled in a postbaccalaureate program to improve her GPA before applying to medical school, she secured a job as a Spanish-English emergency medical scribe in a hospital and worked as a newborn intensive care unit receptionist at the Children's Hospital of Orange County. Rosalva initially struggled to gain access to these shadowing experiences, but these jobs that saw Spanish/English bilingualism as an "in" gave her entry to hospitals and access to patients. As an interpreter at the clinic, she learned how to chart in real time as the provider assessed and examined the patient. She also documented the medical history, physical exam, assessment, results, and treatment plan for them. Rosalva put her Spanish-English bilingual skills to use by interpreting and translating for physicians, collecting data from patients, and shadowing physicians as they assessed, examined, and diagnosed patients. She also secured a "shadow" position at El Centro de Salud de Magdalena in Lima, Perú, where her extended family members lived. Here, she shadowed pediatricians, obstetricians, and family medicine physicians. All of this interpretation labor allowed her to gain a wealth of hands-on experience that strengthened her linguistic capital and application materials.

In his book *Mexican New York*, sociologist Robert C. Smith developed the concept of gendered ethnicity to elucidate how gender helps women acquire more human capital in school and offers them a growing labor market niche in the mainstream economy.[25] Smith also indicates that the consequences of this gendered capital are cumulative. Women stay in school longer or go to better schools, which he hypothesizes precludes their attaching a stigmatized meaning to their ethnicity, gives them better skills, and opens up access to more and better ties beyond their immediate networks. First-generation premedical Latina college students who were bilingual often leveraged their bilingual skills to persist in their premedical and medical school pathways.[26] We also see this with Tanya, Yvette, and Claudia. Tanya secured a position as a research assistant for a School of Optometry as a Spanish translator for a study focused on diabetes and vision. This was her entry point into medicine. Yvette joined a vaccination project helmed by a graduate student in Public Health at UCLA, which gave her access to more medical networks. She went door to door to have Spanish-speaking immigrant families fill out a survey querying them about the vaccination status of children five years old and younger. She was also tasked with organizing health fairs in Los Angeles areas with large Latine immigrant populations such as Compton and Carson. Claudia secured a job as a medical assistant in an underserved clinic in North Philadelphia where the patient base was 90 percent Spanish-speaking. "Of all the providers only one of them was Latina [who] was helping translate for doctors. . . . I started thinking, 'I'm needed here,'" she said. While Spanish/English bilingual skills resulted in more meaningful shadowing opportunities for Latinas, they still had to develop the social networks that they sorely lacked and had a harder time developing them with Latina physicians, who were scarce.

## Panethnic-Based Programs as Empowerment Agents

In the absence of high-status social networks connected to white-collar jobs in their families of origin and access to Latine physicians on college campuses, mentorship hubs such as pan-ethnic medical associations or affinity group programs were necessary for Latina/o physicians, who needed them to connect to mentoring and shadowing opportunities in medical facilities or work-related opportunities in health fields. These programs were not readily available to an older cohort of Latino/a physicians who received their schooling post-Civil Rights, but have sprouted up since then. Organizations such as these played a key supplementary role by providing access to Latine mentors and information. These affinity programs and organizations are usually staffed by co-ethnics and/or bilingual individuals, and they help students and new doctors recognize the value of their cultural and linguistic capital for their careers. Respondents described recognizing that such roots can provide the necessary point of reference to strengthen their self-esteem and aspirations for the future.[27] Latinas, in particular, noted the importance of these organizations to their persistence in becoming doctors. Olivia explained it thus: "No one tells you this game. There [are] a lot of secrets that people don't just open up and then you [find] specific programs that kind of share that information." A pan-ethnic medical organization exposed Olivia to necessary application materials, letter writers, test-taking skills, opportunities to be a clinical volunteer, and access to meaningful research opportunities.

Meeting one person or coming across an affinity program in their undergraduate schooling such as ethnic-themed housing programs or a pan-ethnic medical-based organization during medical school was

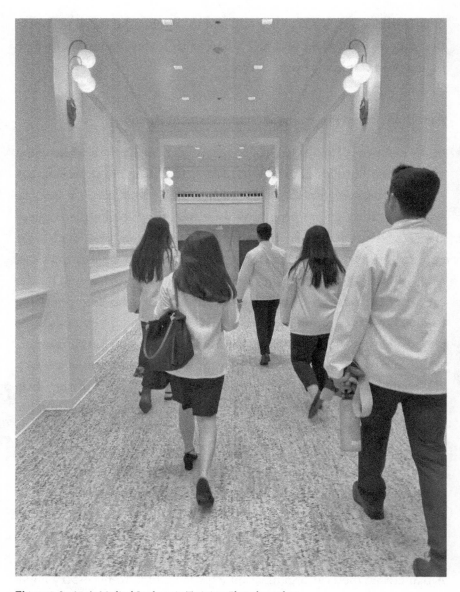

**Figure 3**. Latina/o Medical Students in Training. Photo by author.

transformative. Estebán, in internal medicine, described his experiences with a health-focused organization for Latine students:

> I was lucky that I got as far as I did without a specific mentor. . . . I'm probably more the exception. It's really easy to get off track. . . . I knew I could've used [mentorship] a lot earlier. . . . Things could've probably been a little easier if I knew who to go to. . . . I was part of a group called Los Curanderos [The Healers]. I met other Latinos and then I remember there was a doctor that came to speak to us, and she was positive and motivating. That kind of pushed me to continue during one of those critical points where I was like, 'Maybe it [a career in medicine] was not for me.'

Estebán may have been referring primarily to students who were not first-generation and Latina/o when he suggested that most of his peers had mentors early on, because many respondents said that they had not had mentors until they joined an organization for Latinos/as. Pamela's experience was nearly identical to Estebán's. She said: "If I had the guidance, the mentorship, I would've done better from the beginning. . . . Because [when] I joined CCM [Chican@s/Latin@s for Community Medicine] I met students who had gone through it and that's what helped." She also referenced being exposed to the hidden curriculum, saying that at CCM "I started learning about postbacc programs and things like that." Similarly, Olivia said: "I didn't have mentors at my university, which was unfortunate, but I did have mentors through CCM. The doctors that volunteered their time there, as well as through the summer program at UCLA." Ethnic medical organizations with a focus on pre-medical pathways were crucial for Latina/o doctors who had trouble finding mentors, as many had never met a co-ethnic physician before coming across or joining these organizations.[28]

Laura joined the Latino Medical Student Association, an ethnic organization that highlighted the obstacles and triumphs of Latines interested in medicine, when she began medical school.[29] She said,

In college, I do not think that I had mentorship. . . . [All the advice I got] was more just keep going, keep taking classes. [Not about] what I think I am going to need from medical school. . . . [My undergraduate institution] is such a big school that you kind of get lost in the shuffle. . . . [Finding a mentor] just depends [on] a little bit of luck of meeting the right people and having the right circle.

It was not until her graduate schooling that Laura came across this national organization that served as an umbrella to unify all Latina/o/e medical students.

Respondents' comments align with research showing that social networks with caring and supportive teachers, peers, and school officials can be institutionally produced through academic programs that serve to integrate students, build community, provide access to educational opportunities and institutional knowledge, and foster positive student identities and peer groups.[30] While marginalized students may be able to find and access these supportive educational environments, these institutionally structured social networking groups are rare and may only reach a smaller group of students. They may also only have limited effects when they are mostly run by pre-medical students who rely on each other and provide misguided or ill-informed information.[31]

## "YOU LOOK LIKE COUNTY MATERIAL TO ME": NETWORKED OR PIGEONHOLED INTO PRIMARY CARE?

All physicians are exposed to a range of specialties during rotations during the latter part of medical school, but over half of the Latina/o physicians in the sample specialized in family medicine, internal medicine, or pediatrics. This reflects several factors. First, Latina/o doctors experienced positive effects from training in graduate and postdoctoral programs that had an emphasis on primary care and working with marginalized communities, such as receiving immense gratitude from their poor and immigrant patients as medical students. Second, more recent cohorts had attended medical school programs specifically designed to prepare Latine and non-Latines to work with low-income communities, which encouraged them to work in primary care. Luis, who was of Mexican origin, received a scholarship from the National Service Corps Program.[32] To maintain eligibility his specialty selection was limited to a primary care field in a low-income area, even though he wanted to be a cardiologist. When I asked a Latino faculty member on an admissions committee for such programs about Latine medical students who did not want to work in underserved communities and wanted to work in more affluent areas or seek out higher-paying sub-specialties, he nonchalantly replied, "We usually weed those [applications] out." Third, disadvantage correlates with family medicine. Specifically, Efrain Talamantes and colleagues found that USMGs who attended community college were more likely to train in family medicine than those who never attended community college. They found that among family medicine doctors, 51 percent of Latinos and 42 percent of first-generation college students attended community college, while 32–35 percent of other ethnic groups attended community college.[33] Alejandro said, "There is a tremendous amount of pressure and guilt that is put on Latino doctors to work in poor communities. . . . I'm talking if you don't work in our communities, you're a sellout. . . . There's a pressure to go into primary care."

Respondents were also occupationally tracked into primary care once they became medical residents. Elena, who completed her residency program in the 1970s, only applied to three programs in Los Angeles to fulfill her residency requirements: UCLA, Cedars-Sinai, and Los Angeles County+USC Medical Center, the place that takes the most medically underserved patients. She interviewed at all three. However, her interview with the chairman of a department at Cedars-Sinai Hospital in Los Angeles met an unexpected end. Elena recounted,

I walked into his office in a sad, little suit. My application was sitting in front of him. I sat down, he didn't say anything for a while. He's looking through my CV [moves head back and forth to signal reading] and then he slaps it closed and says, 'You look like county [hospital] material to me.'

At UCLA Elena's treatment was even more blatantly racist and sexist. "[T]he chairman was looking through my application and he goes, 'well, what's this Chicano bullshit say?' [I thought] Oh, you're talking about my commitment to service? Taking care of the same people in this hospital that you have promised to care for? Is that what you're referring to?'" He crumpled her application up and demanded, "Are you planning to get pregnant? I hope you're not going to get married. Are you married? I hope you don't think you're going to get pregnant during residency." "I haven't been thinking about that," Elena responded, confused about what to say in front of this powerful individual since it was "normal at that time" for men to make these misogynistic and discriminatory remarks. Valentina, a Cuban-American doctor, also noted the actionable remarks a world-renowned physician made to her when he called her "*mujercita*" [young lady or little woman] in the operating room as she trained in a San Diego hospital. Because the "culture of medicine" was different back then, as Valentina put it, she did not report it. Elena was open to working with diverse patients of many socioeconomic backgrounds, but she ended up at County/USC. And, instead of pursuing surgery, Valentina found her place as a family medicine practitioner in a low-income free clinic along the border.

There is a long history of Latina/os being tracked in school, with many of them being encouraged to enter vocational jobs or pink-collar work upon high school graduation,[34] and Latina/o physicians experienced this occupational tracking from faculty and higher educational personnel frequently. One Latina physician remembered being told, "You should work with minority communities," by a white physician who had mentored her in her program. The discouragement Luisa experienced came from an institutional agent in a powerful position: "I was discouraged by the dean of my medical school because he said, 'Why do you wanna go into a subspecialty? You said you were interested in primary care?' [Primary care] is what I thought [I wanted to pursue]." But Luisa also discouraged herself to some degree:

> I felt because I was Latina that I had to go into primary care. That is absolutely incorrect. We need Latino physicians in all fields of medicine. . . . I did feel some guilt but my best friend who was also a physician told me that was ridiculous. . . . It makes no sense for people to discourage us from wanting to do some specialties. We should be able to have the freedom to go into anything we want to pursue and not feel bad about it.

She expressed glee that she was in ophthalmology,[35] a field that could benefit from her cultural knowledge as she worked with mostly co-ethnic patients.

Elsa said that she received odd looks from her coworkers when they saw her in their specialty. "When I started the training in gastroenterology there were a few doctors that were like, 'Latino? [She mimicked a confused look.] This is more for overachievers like Chinese or Indian people. What is a Latino doing here compared to the other people?'" Elsa noted that this sentiment went away over time as her coworkers got used to the idea that she was one of them, but she recognized there was a sense that certain specialties were reserved for certain ethnic or racial groups or that members of those groups were better equipped to pursue them.

Gender intersected with ethnicity in these messages. Marisa noted that the feedback she received during her clinical rotations emphasized her interpersonal skills rather than her diagnostic capabilities.

> In my clinical rotations . . . I was given a lot of positive feedback for things that I feel are expected to come from a woman or a Latina. When I was in

the pediatric rotation, they would say, 'Oh, like, you're so good with them [babies]. You're so good with the families, with the moms. You know how to talk. . . .' I got that kind of feedback instead of telling me, 'Oh, your differentials were on point, or your presentation was very well put together.' It was more of the softer feedback, rather than my clinical. [It's] what I was there for. I was, 'Did I diagnose the fever correctly?'

Marisa wanted to know if she was diagnosing symptoms accurately when rendering her assessment of medical conditions. She failed family medicine. She described the reason why:

> Nobody fails family medicine because that's the easiest rotation ever. I managed to fail it because I was with a single white male family medicine doctor in an isolated clinic. It was just me and him for a month. I just couldn't connect. There was nothing for us to talk [about]. It was horrible. That's just my experience with most white [males].

During rotations or their clerkship years, residents are evaluated by preceptors. These evaluations may be subjective and are influenced by social interactions with clinical supervisors and susceptible to racial biases that contribute to grading disparities.[36] Because Marisa was working in an isolated capacity with one physician who did not understand or like how she was communicating with patients, he evaluated her negatively.[37]

Elivet noted another gendered reason for her choice of family medicine. She said that she did not pursue a surgical field because that usually took longer, and she did not want to postpone having a family. "It's more male-dominant. Surgeons are known to have like a rougher attitude. And honestly, I just didn't wanna be in that environment," she elaborated. Another Latina used the masculine refrain *"son más sangrones"* [they are a pain in the neck] to describe surgeons. Joan Cassell notes that "iron surgeons" are trained to have an ethos of "being powerful, invulnerable, untiring."[38] Of the physicians in the sample, eleven worked in a surgical capacity, two worked in "plastics," and three in emergency medicine.

Co-ethnic colleagues could also enforce the norm that Latina/o physicians work in primary care/family medicine and with Latina/o patients. Benito, who worked in family medicine, acknowledged that he had given Latino doctor peers a "hard time" if he felt they were not giving back to the community. He said,

> I see some of my friends that are in other specialties. . . . I sometimes will say, 'Well, are you still feeling connected to what you do? Are you still comfortable in your role of giving back?' Because not every specialty technically will work in an underserved environment. All of us within my circle, wrote [in our] personal statements that we wanted to care for the underserved or worked for our communities. I would hope that they [Latinos in other specialties] can still feel tied to that.

Latina/o physicians explained that they were "programmed" to think that way by their respective training programs. In many ways, Benito also policed and "gave a hard time" to physicians who entered higher-paying specialties to ensure they were still providing for co-ethnics. Kimberly, in emergency medicine, recalled that she completed all of the requirements for family medicine, but changed her focus "last minute," at the end of rotations.

Certainly, there is an enormous need for Latinas/os to receive care from co-ethnic and Spanish-speaking doctors, in every specialty, especially in primary care where there is a critical shortage of doctors that provide more consistent aid.[39] I touch on this in chapter 7. While most Latina/o physicians indicated that they wanted to serve racial/ethnic minority communities and work in specialties that would allow them to have direct daily contact with them, not all of them did. Elena described the high cost of being tracked into serving this population in a system that does not provide the resources for disadvantaged patients that it should. The workload at the county hospital where she was "pigeon-holed" to work by the two other hospitals where she interviewed was prodigious. She described attending the births of over a hundred babies in one twenty-four-hour shift. Noting it was one of the worst days of her life, she said, "That's about the same number some places do in a month. We did that in one day! I was responsible for all those women and their outcomes even though I was not a faculty member." The doctors, nurses, and other health-care professionals she was supervising were culturally inexperienced and the workload was relentless.

### "You're a Sellout": Rotations and Specialty Selection

Lorenzo addressed the question Benito described immediately at the beginning of our interview. He worked in a glamorous office building with a colorful fish tank in the lobby. A tall man with thick, black-rimmed glasses, Lorenzo had an assortment of plaques in his office, highlighting his many accomplishments. "So, are you here to find out how I rationalize going into plastic surgery versus helping out the community?" he said as soon as I sat down.

It was not my first question, but I answered, "I was going to ask you about specialty selection."

As he moved the mouse to close the windows on his computer he explained, "In surgery, you still help out the community in different ways. There is less of a stigma for Latinos to [specialize] in surgery today. It's becoming more acceptable." Lorenzo indicated that he debated between going into oral surgery or cardiothoracic surgery. However, he ultimately selected reconstructive surgery because he was thinking about his future lifestyle. At some point in his life, he wanted a wife and children, and this specialty would give him the flexibility to do that.

Lorenzo had experienced resistance to pursuing a specialty that did not connote service to the larger Latino community. He recounted that when he was asked to give a talk at a prominent Latino ethnic medical organization, the first question he asked the audience was, "'What place does a reconstructive surgeon have in your organization? And what do people think about plastic surgery?'" Somebody in the audience immediately yelled, "Sellout!" Lorenzo was perturbed that people considered him a "sellout," especially co-ethnics, and he noted that while most of his work is cosmetic surgeries, the resulting income allowed him to help his Mexican immigrant mother and sister financially. It also supported pro bono work that is more meaningful. He explained that he helped out the community by doing reconstructive surgery for cancer patients. While being a surgeon involves occupational prestige, more so than doctors in family medicine because of the extra years of schooling necessary and the higher salary, surgeons dealt with additional pressures not expressed by those who worked in family medicine.

Understanding the mechanisms behind specialty selection for Latina/o physicians is important given their low representation in the field overall. Unlike white physicians, they face a presumption that they will "give back" to the community. Most of them do, but this is an added element that racial/ethnic minority professionals from working-class origins who enter the middle class carry and negotiate.[40]

Alicia noted that other co-ethnic doctors would call her either the Princess of Pasadena or a "sellout" because she had transitioned half-time to a concierge practice, which meant she did not work with insurance and charged her patients a retainer/concierge fee. This meant that a lot of her patients were much more affluent, and some were millionaires. She said,

A lot of Latino doctors said to me, 'Alicia, you're a sellout. Why would you want to be working in Pasadena with all these very wealthy people?' . . . I said, 'All of you are missing the boat. Pasadena is located in a very wealthy area, but we are surrounded by Highland Park, Boyle Heights, Eagle Rock, and North Pasadena, which is primarily low-income. Patients come to me from a lot of places. How lovely to be in a community where I could promote Latino health and I could admit patients to a hospital that is five stars, where they now get admitted to a place where they will benefit from the best services?'

Alicia saw offering concierge services as a vital measure so that she could balance being a mother and a doctor, provide scholarships to the community, and provide better access and service to low-income groups. However, she received pushback from mentors and other co-ethnic physicians for branching away from solely offering primary care in marginalized communities.

Becoming a doctor is not solely about being smart, but it is about having the right social capital networks in the absence of ample familial and educational resources provided by socioeconomic status. Individual perseverance alone is not sufficient to succeed in predominantly white and heteromasculine fields,[41] and in this chapter I focus on the various ways that Latina/o physicians sought mentorship hubs to attain the meaningful training opportunities that they needed to get ahead, as well as how the intersection of gender and ethnicity affected their opportunity structures as they selected their specialties. In their efforts to find a supportive hub, they came across gatekeeping, institutional, and empowerment agents or organizations. While one might assume that Latina/o physicians found support from co-ethnic mentors in STEM, most Latina/o doctors described them as few and far between. Instead, the interviews suggest that more recent cohorts of Latina/o physicians found stronger support networks from pan-ethnic associations or smaller inclusion programs on their college campuses that saw their ethnic and linguistic capital as an asset. These pan-ethnic organizations do not open the floodgates, but they do create small apertures and serve as a bulwark from the institutionalized discrimination that they and the older cohort of physicians experienced.

Universities across the nation have fluctuated in their support of diversity efforts by either supporting or dismantling affirmative action efforts, or, more recently leaning into diversity, equity, and inclusion and Hispanic Serving Institution (HSI) funding efforts, but I suggest that organizations are still trying to catch up in the development of initiatives to encourage the retention of women and underrepresented groups in STEM. Their efficacy is mixed as some scholars demonstrate the various ways organizational inertia manifests at the everyday granular level.[42] USMG Latina/o doctors mention this, too.

First-generation college students had significant trouble securing meaningful shadowing experiences, but Spanish/English linguistic capital helped women access a gendered network where they were able to leverage their bilingual skills to gain access to meaningful experiences with patients. Men, on the other hand, faced significant challenges and often racialized slights until they met a really significant other who could use the weight of their credentials to create apertures and opportunities for them. They interpreted these connections as serendipitous, but they were also "found" after multiple attempts. Larger gendered and ethnic stereotypes of Latinidad, however, restricted and pigeonholed them into certain specialties. In many ways, the sorting process steered those who made it through all the hoops and hurdles into family and internal medicine. Most of the doctors I spoke with are content with these specialties, but others lamented the disadvantages of not being able to diversify into other specialties. It is unfair and racist to track people into certain specialties because of their ethnicity, as their future mobility may be compromised in the long run. Over time, and as they move up in the medical hierarchy, however, men physicians experience a gender advantage over Latina doctors.

In the next chapter, I examine how gender-based discrimination produces markedly different experiences on the job for Latina/o physicians, with Spanish skills leading to bilingual women having fuller plates than their co-ethnic male colleagues after they move up in the medical hierarchy to the fully licensed practitioner stage.

# 5.

# GENDERED DEFERENCE OR SABOTAGE?

"It was like God came into the room when a white male Caucasian doctor showed up. It was like 'Lisa, go get the doctor some food.'"

—LISA MACIAS, Family Medicine

"Women unfortunately don't treat women well [in medicine]. . . . They're more afraid of men [and] absolutely show more respect."

—ALICIA PARRA, Internal Medicine

MY BROTHER, A DENTIST, saw Lisa give a presentation at a Latino Medical School Association (LMSA) conference, and he asked her if he could share her contact information with me. I met her and her teenage niece, who wanted to hear the conversation because she is an aspiring Latina doctor herself, at a coffee shop in Southern California in the evening. A 1.5 generation Spanish/English bilingual Salvadoran doctor, she completed a portion of her residency in Perú, and she had just returned from there to work at the small clinic near the coffee shop where she had "matched." Lisa explained that she

Portions of the chapter are related to a previously published article: Flores, Glenda M. and Maricela Bañuelos. 2021. "Gendered Deference: Perceptions of Authority and Competency Among Latina/o Physicians." *Gender & Society* 35: 110–35.

had been able to get credit for the time in Perú, although she had to pay her expenses out of her pocket. In Perú she worked in different places such as orphanages with small children. There she worked alongside a younger Peruvian male physician who oversaw a small clinic.

Initially, Lisa thought, "Cool, he's treating me normally." She felt that she and the young Peruvian doctor were on equal planes, tending to patients together. But when a white American physician arrived to volunteer there as well, that all changed. The Peruvian doctor began to expect her to assist him. Whereas they had shared taxis when she first started to ensure she arrived at the correct location, he stopped being willing to share the fare with her. He would tell her to take money from the counter and buy him fruit. Lisa said, "I was like 'What happened?' I didn't care. I can find my way. . . . But I [could not] believe it was different. I thought maybe it was just because we are all volunteers?"

Lisa reasoned that perhaps the Peruvian doctor "did not have a picture" of all the volunteers and forgot that she was a doctor, too. She was assigned to see patients who wanted help from her rather than from the white American physician. She was expected to interpret for the white doctor, who could not fully communicate with his patients. She was exasperated recalling the experience:

> I ended up doing way more [work] than that [white] doctor! That doctor slowed me down because his Spanish was broken and he did not know anything about medical Spanish, which I had been studying. They were using me to interpret [for him] and I was mad . . . because there are so many patients to see and instead of being doctors [plural], we're almost like one doctor because I have to stop with my patient, go [to his], and interpret. 'Why am I doing that?'

Lisa seemed to manage her emotions as she went on,

> I am okay doing it [interpreting], but it was just funny that [another] Latino [doctor], a Peruvian guy, was putting him [the white doctor] on a pedestal because he is male, white, older, and I am the opposite.

Lisa thought it was peculiar that a fellow Latino doctor would treat her as inferior to a white male doctor who was less capable of communicating with his patients and of being an effective doctor.

Displays of deference and respect, such as the ones the Peruvian doctor showed to the white volunteer, were gendered and affected Latina physicians' self-presentation as well. In this chapter, I examine how gender shapes perceptions of authority and competence for Latina/o doctors in part through what I call *gendered deference* dynamics. I argue that everyone—from physicians to nurses and staff to patients—is complicit in maintaining this inequality across the medical education pipeline and into the profession. I take an intra-Latina/o dynamics lens to show how gendered deference and racism manifests for doctors via three main themes: 1) gendered cultural taxation; 2) microaggressions from women nurses and staff; and 3) the questioning of authority and competence. These processes frequently result in unequal outcomes for Latina physicians as they move up vertically in the doctor hierarchy. They are routinely over-included in job tasks and allotted fewer resources to do their work. Interestingly, the bilingual abilities that were perceived as assets for Latinas during training as apprentices become invisibilized as they move up the medical hierarchy. Co-ethnic male doctors perpetuated this hierarchy as they blamed their Latina colleagues for the gendered microaggressions they experienced from nurses and staff. Moreover, Latina doctors are forced to accept gender-biased treatment to provide their patients with equitable health care. Age and the high social status accorded to doctors, in general, act as a salve that buffers some of these gendered microaggressions over their career span.

## UNDERSTANDING GENDERED DEFERENCE AND DEMEANOR IN ORGANIZATIONS

All organizations, especially medical ones, have "inequality regimes" that maintain class, gender, and racial hierarchies that are not always visible to all members of society.[1] They operate by fluid dynamics that may change depending on the type of organization, the characteristics of the people who work there, and the job tasks. While the STEM fields are presumed to be "neutral" and to have no distinguishable organizational culture or identity, there are racist and sexist ideologies embedded within the social structure that become hegemonic, giving workers the sense that they need to manipulate their bodies or relegate their cultural identities to the margins to avoid prejudice. Femininity is often perceived as antithetical to a scientist's identity, and women may attempt to embody masculine forms to gain respect. To do so they may change the style and content of their speech, posture, clothing, hair length, and body shape.[2]

I build on sociologist Erving Goffman's ideas of deference and demeanor to elucidate how gendered displays of deference and demeanor, or lack thereof, shape the white coat's multivalence for Latina and Latino doctors. In the Americas, doctors occupy a higher position in the organizational structure of the medical field than nurses and staff. Goffman notes that "doctors give medical orders to nurses, but nurses do not give medical orders to doctors. . . . [I]n some hospitals in America nurses stand up when a doctor enters the room, but doctors do not ordinarily stand up when nurses enter the room."[3] He explains two modes of presentation rules that conduct falls into: *deference acts* and *demeanor acts*. Deference acts encompass presentational and interpersonal rituals that specify what should be done and how recipients should be treated in interactions. These may be linguistic statements of praise or depreciation, gestural, or spatial (such as preceding others through doors), or task-embedded.

Demeanor, on the other hand, is an individual's outward behavior, displayed through actions, facial expressions, the way people talk, or the presentation of self. A well-mannered person has discretion and sincerity, modesty in claims regarding self, command of speech, and self-control over emotions and appetites. These displays of deference and demeanor accentuate or highlight the inherent status differentials embedded in medicine.[4] In what follows, I unpack the components of my concept of *gendered deference* by focusing on interpersonal interactions that occur daily to demonstrate my overarching argument that the white coat's polyvalence is not dispersed equally within Latinidad, exposing men and women to different forms of gendered racism. The overall result systematically penalizes bilingual Latina doctors.

## GENDERED CULTURAL TAXATION

Latina/o physicians explained that their Spanish/English bilingual and bicultural abilities were assets in their jobs, but they often felt burdened by translation demands, with women having to shoulder this aspect of the job more often than men. Latina/o physicians noted Spanish/English bilingualism often meant they performed tasks outside the bounds of their job description for doctors and staff across facilities. Thalia, an internal medicine doctor, elucidates this pattern:

> I sent [a patient] to the GI [gastroenterology] specialist, and they saw her and did all of these tests. She comes and sees me about a month later. I ask her, '*Señora Gutierrez, ¿qué le dijieron, qué entiende usted porque tiene cirrosis?*' *Y ella me dice, 'Pues yo no se.' Y le dije, '¿Cómo que no sabe? ¿Qué no fue al especialista? ¿Pues qué le explicaron?' Y ella dice, 'No pues nada, que es usted me iba a explicar todo.'* ['Ms. Gutierrez, what did they tell you? What do you understand about having cirrhosis?' And she tells me, 'I don't know.' I tell her, 'How come you don't know? Didn't you go to the specialist? What did he explain to you?' And she tells me, 'No, nothing. That you were going to explain everything to me']. So, I took a deep breath and said, '*¿yo?*' [me?] *La señora dijo, 'si porque usted es mi doctora y me va a decir todo lo que esta pasando.'* [The patient said, 'Yes because you are my doctor and were going to tell me everything that was happening.'] There are very few things that irk me and that is one of them. . . . And it's not that I can't [interpret]. I am capable of doing that, but I'm not the specialist and you just saw them, and

I think it's their absolute responsibility to explain to [the patients] in a way that they understand or get a translator.

Minority professionals are often tasked with performing cultural competence and sensitivity when working with co-ethnics or co-racials, an example of what Amado Padilla terms "cultural taxation" and Adia Harvey Wingfield terms "equity work."[5] Wingfield describes "racial outsourcing," in which Black physicians and nurses perform additional job tasks not asked of white counterparts when serving racial or language minority populations. Thalia was "fully capable" of translating the results for the patient, but she nonetheless resented the specialist's abdication of their obligation to explain to the patient in a way that the patient understood, even if that required an interpreter. Specialists from other facilities frequently failed to provide interpretations to Spanish-speaking immigrant patients and instead relied on referring bilingual doctors to do their work.

This unremunerated effort is heavily gendered in medicine. Yvette, who worked in pediatric medicine, explained the different workloads between her male colleagues and herself related to her linguistic abilities. She said in one month she saw over "one hundred patients" while her white male and monolingual English colleague saw "a little above forty." She explained, "I haven't looked [at the schedule] recently, but one day, I happened to look through their schedules and one of them saw five, one of them saw seven, one of them saw three, and one of them saw twelve. I was very upset." Clinics need Latina/o physicians, but Yvette emphasized the cultural exploitation at the workplace and noticed monolingual English-speaking doctors relied on her uncompensated bilingual labor to explain to every Spanish-speaking patient what was going on with their health. Indeed, sociologist Joya Misra and colleagues explain that exploitation at the workplace occurs when more powerful actors benefit at the expense of the less powerful, appropriating scarce resources including unpaid labor.[6]

Bilingual Latina doctors who opened their own practices found that cultural taxation subsumed the occupational hierarchy that might otherwise have put them above staff and nurses. I observed an interaction in which a white medical assistant wearing a headset said *"un momento"* into the microphone. Perla, the Puerto Rican doctor who owned the practice, heard the words, and she immediately grabbed a headset and answered the call. *"Hola soy la doctora. Tengo disponible a las doce. Perfecto."* [Hello, I'm the doctor. Noon is available. Perfect!]," then, to the assistant, Tessa, "I'll put her here." She put the visit into the computer system. It seemed like Tessa was not well-equipped to help patients on days when Perla's Mexican American husband, who served as the bilingual clinic manager, was absent.

Latina physicians explained that linguistic competence meant that patients had higher expectations of them. Janet, in family medicine, explained that her bilingualism meant that Spanish-speaking patients expected more out of her because they had finally found someone who could speak their language. "They're going to tell me there are ten issues and they want me to address all of them," Janet declared. While patients' willingness to tell Janet about their problems suggests that she gave them more comprehensive care than her colleagues, facing higher expectations in the US health-care context where physicians are expected to maximize their billing enacts a gendered cultural tax that colleagues without Spanish competence did not face.

Other Latina physicians noted the frequency with which they provided interpretation services for nurses. Laura, in family medicine, explained:

> A lot of my patients complain. I will tell them, 'You have to get this lab test. My nurse will come back and explain to you how to get that test.' It is really hard if she cannot communicate with them. She has to grab another nurse or somebody else to help her out. Or I have to do it. So, it falls back on me. It is a struggle that I am ready to deal with. It is not new.

Laura realized that she was fully capable of doing this and generally did not mind performing this work; however, it added to her already heavy workload. While doctors recognized that the practice was unfair, they saw no point in complaining about it because they realized that medical institutions were not seeking to expand these resources.

Unlike the South Asian women physicians in Lata Murti's study who experienced social marginalization and exclusion from their coworkers,[7] Latina physicians were not socially marginalized per se, but instead were repeatedly and regularly pulled in by various parties to provide their linguistic capital and cultural competency and rarely received extra compensation or recognition for this skill from their coworkers. They were over-included in these job tasks because they were bilingual women. Bilingual and bicultural Latina doctors were expected to perform Spanish/English interpreting work at all times, and when they said "no" or explained that it wasn't their job, they would receive a hostile response or an accusation that they were difficult to work with. Male doctors experienced the expectation that they would interpret too, but their interview comments suggest that they could resist without significant negative repercussions. Jacob, in internal medicine, commented,

> I'm generally happy to [interpret]. It's unique though . . . a more common thing is to grab the nearest nurse that speaks Spanish. The patients comprehend that that's why the nurse is in the room. It's strange when I get pulled in. . . . It's much more common that people will grab the nurse though.

Jacob's colleagues wanted him to interpret when it was convenient for them, but such cases were not very common. He "had to say" that it was "strange" to be treated in a way unsuited to his stature as a doctor, but he did not report any problems with having made this objection.

Another source of gendered cultural taxation was that women patients often preferred to see women doctors, a pattern several respondents observed. Laura explained how it compounded the cultural tax for her: "[A] lot of time they request a female doctor if they're female. A lot of times, if they're Spanish-speaking they will request a Spanish-speaking physician." Latina doctors noted that Latina patients felt greater cultural, emotional, and physical comfort with Latina physicians than with co-ethnic male doctors. Raquel, an internal medicine doctor, expressed her frustration at having to see more patients than her male colleagues but also understood why. She explained,

> [Latina patients] don't want to be examined by male doctors. I get all of those. Which, excuse me, they're doctors too! Why do I have to see them when they're not my patients for the breast exam? The pelvic? For vaginal discharge? All of those female-related things? 'I'm anxious, I'm depressed'. . . . [T]hey feel males don't listen to their mental health issues. That's probably true because men will be like, 'Tough it out'. . . . They think we're more compassionate.

Mental health issues are sometimes stigmatized in Latine cultures,[8] which may be part of the reason Raquel expected her male colleagues to voice such opinions.

Elivet had similar experiences:

> We [women doctors] are requested more. We'll have the same number of patients on our schedule, male providers and female providers, but they will request us if there's any gynecological issue. They will ask us if it's more of an anxiety/depression issue. We get more work in that sense. I don't know if this is a different expectation or a different dynamic because we are expected to do the same things as our male colleagues. Sometimes, we do more because we see more patients and different kinds of patients that require more attention.

Latino physicians generally acknowledged that because patients preferred women doctors, Latina doctors saw more Latine patients than they did, and a few even claimed they saw no more patients than white doctors. However, much like Latina doctors, they felt that they were expected to provide more services to Latine patients than white doctors were. For instance, Ignacio, a family medicine physician, described how he had to treat more severe conditions while seeing patients due to the lack of culturally competent doctors and lack of health-care accessibility for low-income Latine patients. He said,

> People come in with a big list. They expect you to cure their thirty years of problems in a twenty-minute visit. That can't be done. Latinos tend to hold a lot in, and then when they come to see you, 'Oh doctor, mire tengo estas preguntas' [Oh doctor, look I have these questions] and then they have twenty questions. . . . Or, say they just got insurance for the first time, and they've never seen a doctor and now they have all these chronic and vast diseases that should have never gotten [so bad].

Such experience constituted labor other doctors frequently did not have to perform.

Some participants expressed discontent with their colleagues or workplaces for refusing to recognize the importance of culturally competent patient care, a topic I explore in greater detail in chapter 7. Laura explained that she was in the process of convincing the nurse manager who supervises nurses in her clinic that they needed a Spanish-speaking nurse on staff. She said,

> Right now, I am trying to make a point that I need a Spanish-speaking nurse in my clinic. The nurse manager does not think that I necessarily need a Spanish-speaking nurse. I made it a case that my patients are all Spanish-speaking or the majority are and that it would be beneficial to them if I had a Spanish-speaking nurse because they could communicate with my nurse things that I do not have time for. It just brought out the fact that I feel she does not understand what it's like to go to a doctor and not be able to communicate. She has no idea what that means.

These discussions between Laura and the nurse manager were ongoing and happened frequently, with no resolution on the horizon. At one point the nurse manager replied, "I did not even know you had that many Spanish-speaking patients," failing to recognize the demographic and linguistic characteristics of the patient population.

Such experiences contrast with those in research that focuses on white women. Lauren Alfrey and France Winddance Twine found that supervisors rewarded LGBTQ+ white women programmers, technical writers, and engineers who presented as genderfluid for their competence and interpersonal skills when they did not present as conventionally feminine.[9] In a related vein, sociologist Sharla Alegria explains that interpersonal skills offered white women who worked in the production, design, or maintenance of computer hardware, software, or networks a "step-stool" that helped them gain slight advancement in the tech fields.[10]

By contrast, Raquel's assumption that speaking Spanish gave her an advantage in serving Spanish-speaking patients produced hostility. She recounted,

> When I said, 'I'm so happy to work in [this city]; there's a lot of Spanish-speaking patients.' He [an Asian doctor/colleague] said, 'Well before you came, we were doing fine without you. We have this thing. Have you ever heard of it? It's a translator line. So, we don't need Spanish speakers. We got this box, and they could speak their language.'

Latina/o doctors like Raquel reported that their cultural competence allowed them to foster trust, practice mannerisms that denote respect, understand cultural beliefs and taboos related to health, and know common homemade *remedios* [remedies], all of which allowed them to better advise Latines on health-related matters. Gender inequality manifested itself in different ways, and bilingual Latinas working in the "token" context or as the "lonely only" had more of the workload pushed in their direction.[11]

## DEFERENCE OR SABOTAGE? MICROAGGRESSIONS FROM WOMEN NURSES AND STAFF

Male physicians had a distinct gender advantage over Latina physicians when it came to receiving symbolic displays of deference and respect from women nurses and staff, both Latine and non-Latine. Relationships between women nurses and staff and Latina/o physicians in the workplace fell into two categories: deference or sabotage. Fausto, who specialized in pediatrics, noted that he and two other men in his medical program would rarely have to do tasks such as drawing blood from patients because women nurses were quick to offer to do it for them. Chuckling, Fausto remarked,

> We [the men in my program] joked we would never have to draw blood or anything. We did draw blood. But looking back on the number of times I had to versus my female colleagues had to, was a little different. [Latinas] had [to draw blood] way more [than us] because the nurses would offer all the time. It clearly came down to gender. I told [female colleagues] I think it was how nice I was. I would talk to [the nurses and say] I couldn't draw blood . . . not in a manipulative way but I felt like I could. They [women physicians] just felt like they couldn't do that.

Fausto described two dynamics here: nurses assuming they should do part of his job for him, and women colleagues feeling less comfortable asking for help.

Jacob described a different dynamic. While less than 5 percent of registered nurses are of Latina/o backgrounds,[12] he worked with many Latina nurses, and he said that he found it made it easier to develop close relationships with Latina nurses if he spoke Spanish to them, a tactic he described thus: "A lot of the nurses are Hispanic and it's cheating, but it works. Like [a] way to get in with the nurses is to start talking in Spanish. It was instantaneous." Bilingual Latino men recognized they were able to use their linguistic capital to get women to perform tasks for them to make their workdays run more smoothly.

Mariano, a pediatric surgeon, noted that Latina nurses and staff often performed small interpersonal acts of deference toward him, and he also felt that speaking Spanish had made this more likely:

> I was lucky. . . . I wasn't expected to do anything. I could just do whatever I wanted because I was a male and [spoke] Spanish. . . . It was amazing! If I had a charge nurse who was Mexican, I [would] get special treatment. It's really interesting. I mean, they'd look out for me and if there was a potluck or something, they always made me a plate and the other guy standing around would say, 'Hey, where did you get the plate from?'

Mariano marveled at the fact that, because of his gender and linguistic abilities, in conjunction with being a surgeon, Latina nurses and staff would go out of their way to cater to him over Latina doctors and other white, non-Latine physicians.[13] According to the 2017 National Nursing Workforce Survey, registered nurses are overwhelmingly women (90.9 percent). It was women nurses and the staff's discriminatory practices that upheld and perpetuated this gender advantage for bilingual Latino men and pushed them up higher in the medical hierarchy over Latinas.

Anthropologist Joan Cassell found that women nurses were deferential to older men surgeons and not to women surgeons. The white women in her study who had more recently gained entry were frequently questioned about their expertise and expected to modify their behaviors in the operating room. Age intersected with gender, causing nurses to act as "enforcers of gender-appropriate behavior"[14] who engaged in same-sex policing by helping male surgeons with gowns and gloves before operations while women surgeons dressed themselves. Nurses and coworkers perpetuated a discriminatory gender order[15] because the gendered job queue was in the initial stages of shifting status beliefs about gender.[16]

## Status Beliefs

Naturally, gender intersected with the esteem and respect accorded to high-status Latinas/os, as men were regularly allotted more resources to fulfill their duties. Sociologist Cecilia Ridgeway notes that cultural status beliefs about which group is "better" can generate material advantages for certain groups.[17] Cultural status beliefs can also bias evaluations of competence and evoke associational preference biases. Associational preference biases shape who people form ties with and favor to gain opportunities or affection. The interactions of Miguel Nuñez, an orthopedic surgeon, and the women he employed in his private practice illustrate this process. I found that Latina staff in his private practice addressed him as Dr. Nuñez while he addressed them by their first names, even those who were older than him. He seemed to have a pleasant relationship with them; when he was giving me a tour of his practice, he indicated that some of his employees had been working for him for thirty years and that he had a good working relationship with them. "Am I a good boss?" Miguel yelled out as one of the Latina staff members walked out of his office. "The best boss ever!" the woman yelled back. Miguel showed me the file she had left for him. It was a list of his cases for the following day with a Post-it that read, "Good afternoon, Dr. Nuñez" with a happy face.

Latino physicians played into these cultural status beliefs at the everyday actor level. They used the word "cattiness" to describe women's interactions with nurses. Latinas, on the other hand, felt that nurses would perform small acts of sabotage toward Latina doctors. Janet described the problem this way: "I think when it comes to many nurses (males or females), they kind of don't like taking orders from you. Who are you to give me an order?" Latina physicians tried different strategies such as bringing nurses sweets or helping them around the office to gain favor, but it rarely worked.

Alicia, an internal medicine doctor, echoed these interactions by individual actors. "I get along with the nurses, but I know if a man walks into the hospital and says, 'Where's the labs of this patient?' The nurses go, 'What do you need?' I could have been asking that nurse the same question and it would have taken her an hour." Alicia said that sometimes nurses tell her to wait because the male doctor "always screams"—that is, yells at them if they are not prompt. She internally responds, "It's not that he yells or screams. It's because he's a man and you have more respect for him. You don't realize your underlying bias because nobody is calling you out on it." By Alicia's account, she gets along with the nurses in part because she does not say this part out loud. Her experience aligns with a description of the dynamics between doctors and nurses at an urban, university-based hospital in Canada: "Nurses were more willing to serve and defer to male physicians. They approached female physicians on a more egalitarian basis, were more comfortable communicating with them, yet more hostile toward them."[18]

Elivet reported similar experiences. She noted,

> When it comes to little favors or whatever, [nurses and staff] ask the female providers to do the extra work. Let's say a patient shows up late and their doctor won't see them. They're more likely to ask the female providers, and I know this is true not just of me but my female coworkers, they're more likely to ask us, 'Will you see this patient?' . . . So, I don't know if they feel more intimidated by the males or they just feel like there's more indifference by the males, but they'll try to avoid giving them as much work as us.

When nurses were deferential to men, Latinas paid the price. A curious feminist intersectional lens is useful here, as it reflects how women respond to their positioning in a society that privileges men, especially white men. Nurses expect other actors in their organizations to judge them according to these beliefs of the gender (and racial) hierarchy in medicine, and they must take status beliefs into account in their behavior, whether or not they personally endorse them, to constrain high-status women of color doctors. This interference may not have been intentional, as women nurses did not behave this way to be treated better in the workplace or to gain favor from men doctors. However, they know that men in medicine hold the power, and they do not want to be the recipients of their outbursts, which could affect their job security and mobility. Their small self-preservation tactics cause a type of collateral damage that systematically sabotages Latina doctors.

Unlike male physicians, Latina physicians emphasized that nurses, both Latine and non-Latine, would consciously or subconsciously engage in subtle acts of sabotage to undermine their efforts at work. These acts of sabotage took different forms, with some of them falling under status bias—such as when Latina doctors noticed nurses took "forever" to complete a simple task they requested for a patient while doing it much faster for a male physician. "Nurses were mean to me. . . . They were particularly not happy to have a Latina doctor," Gloria said. More than one Latina physician in the study described it as a "female screwing another female." Perla explained, "Nurses are far more likely to question your judgment, especially if you're a new doctor. But they do it in such a rude way a lot of the time . . . the dynamic there could be a little bit tough." To avoid working with Latina medical assistants who dismissed her instructions or took a long time to administer injections to patients when she worked in facilities in downtown Los Angeles and South Central LA, Perla saved up to open her private practice. Rather than exerting their power over their less status-privileged coworkers, Perla and other Latina physicians would routinely endure the inequities caused by these cross-category interactions and were forced to begrudgingly participate in their durability.

Elivet, a family medicine doctor who worked for a large HMO, noted the implicit salience of these patterns too, especially when a chaperone[19] was in the room with her and a patient. She explained,

"The males have chaperones for every female exam all the time. We [women] don't because we're busier and, even if we do, the assistant will come into our room, and she'll just stand in the corner and be there as an observer. But if she's assisting the male provider, she's handing him the equipment." Not only did Latina physicians see more patients overall, but they also performed tasks that assistants would automatically do for men. Vicki echoed Elivet's sentiments that nurses and staff were deferential to men. She said,

> I was on-call in the hospital. . . . [and] I asked the RN, 'Do you know where [Max] is?' and she says, 'Well that's something you can figure out.' So, she gave me attitude. . . . [W]hat struck me is I've seen this RN interact with white male doctors, and she would never speak to them like that. At that moment I felt like, I don't know if she knows I'm a doctor . . . because I'm female, because I'm Latina, like it's not important. . . . I've personally seen this RN. You know? The sixty-year-old white female. A male doctor comes in, 'Oh, doctor, what do you need? Here's your stuff.'

Isabel was promoted to a traditionally male role in the hospital where she worked, the chief of her section, and she faced gendered racism from support staff. She said:

> The secretaries had a hard time accepting that I was a new chief. She [a particular secretary] had worked for the previous chief of the section of pediatric radiology and he became the chairman of the section and then I became the section chief. She just couldn't take it and ended up leaving. . . . One time she was just like, 'I'm having a really hard time accepting you as my chief.'

At times men physicians noticed the microaggressions Latinas faced, but sometimes blamed them for the actions of nurses and others, failing to recognize their gender privilege. Rather than advocating for Latina physicians when they faced status challenges and resistance from lower-ranked people at work, men blamed them for these interpersonal interactions by relying on the cultural frame of gender. For example, Esteban, an internal medicine physician, remarked, "One of the female docs was complaining. They take things personally. I don't know why or how, but there sometimes can be more of a clash among females." Latino doctors relished the small acts of gendered deference they received from staff and nurses, which encouraged them to feel that when nurses and Latina doctors "bumped heads" it was based on "personality" issues instead of a discriminatory gender order that pushed them up at work. Enrique brought baked goods his mother provided to him while he was living with her during his medical residency to win favor with nurses—a form of opportunity hoarding. However, Latina doctors who tried this strategy felt it was ineffective. For example, Luisa worked in a practice where she was the only woman, and the rest of the doctors were Asian men. They frequently asked her for favors, such as taking their on-call shifts, but when she asked one man, who repeatedly asked her for help, to cover hers, he replied, "How could you think that I would do that for you?" Luisa thought that there was a culture of collaboration and reciprocity in her job, where if someone asked for help or a favor, it would be repaid later. However, she soon realized that she was expected to help or could be asked for favors without them being returned. Ultimately, Luisa had put her "foot down" and ceased the practice altogether because it was creating problems for her.

Several Latino physicians told me nurses respected them more than their women counterparts because they were "nice" and treated nurses as important team members, even though the deference they received often involved nurses repeatedly performing tasks for men physicians they could have easily done themselves. Latino doctors benefited from the racialized sexism and microaggressions that Latina physicians experienced.[20]

## Modifying Self-Presentation

Some Latina physicians mentioned they tried to "act like men" or "talk like men" to gain more respect. Rocío had been told to speak with a lower and deeper voice at a professional training in order to be taken seriously. Yvette said that she felt particular pressure to appear more masculine because she is a pediatrician, and that she tried to walk more like a man. Gender and work sociologists Gladys García-López and Denise Segura found a similar trend among Latina lawyers, who attempted to modify their comportment in front of judges and were mindful of their wardrobes, especially in the courtroom.[21] Yvette described her reasons thus:

> People feel like peds [short for pediatrics] is touchy-feely and newborn babies. I feel like in peds you still need to assert yourself and other people in other specialties may feel like, 'Oh, you're not tough enough to play with the boys.' I know I remember in one of my orthopedics orientations there were these big, tall, men. They had big legs and walked like this [motions a long and fast stride]. I am like 'Oh, okay. I have to be just like them. I have to play'. . . . Some people may not think you have the capability because of your ethnic background but you just kind of have to say I don't care about what you think.

Luisa explained how she modified her personality to address the disrespect she received when her coworkers would move her scheduled time in the operating room without giving her advance notice. While Luisa explained that the nurses who worked with her treated her well, they would take away her time or let another doctor replace her appointments. When this would happen, she felt compelled to fight for her patients and said they "would never do that to my male colleague!" She explained,

> [Asian and white men doctors] think, I should be nicer or, they think they can get away with things the males would never tolerate. . . . I find myself making up for that sometimes where I have to be a little bit more serious or sterner. I voice my opinion so people don't think they can push me aside.

Latina doctors tried to change their self-presentation to adopt more masculine traits and avoid traits typically associated with femininity, for example, being kind, nurturing, or accommodating.

Yet, being assertive on the job could cause trouble. If she didn't "say something the right way," other women Janet worked with would "make a big fuss about it." Indeed, studies show that women who self-promote, act assertively, or dominate interactions are more negatively evaluated. Lucito, who considered himself an ally to women providers in family medicine, described them as "inflexible." Fernando, a surgeon and another self-described ally to women physicians, was aware of the difficulties Latinas faced. At the same time, he was relieved that he did not have to face them: "If you're too manly then you're just trying to be one of the guys. If you act too much like a woman then you will never fit in. I'm happy I don't have to go through it." Virginia Valian explains the catch-22 thus: "A "feminine woman runs the risk of seeming less competent; the more she typifies the schema for a woman, the less she matches the schema for the successful professional. . . . A woman with masculine traits runs the risk of appearing unnatural and deviant."[22] Thalia, who is in private practice, noted that being assertive to get the results she wanted from staff was a source of conflict. She felt her staff thought that as a Latina she would be "more patient," "open," and relax her expectations of staff members who would "take more time" to follow through on her requests than a man or a white person.

It's a hindrance if I am assertive. They see that as negative. My nurse will tell me [that] when she's off nobody wants to work with me [laughs]. *Es porque soy exigente* [it's because I'm demanding] and it's not any different than being a male, right? . . . I want you to do your job. . . . I have high expectations because you [nurses and office staff] represent me, and the practice represents me. Everything represents me as the ultimate deliverer of services. I would like to think that you are going to be as proud of that as I am.

Thalia explained that she recognized staff might have an "off day," but she would "call them out" if she had to ask repeatedly. "I'm not the person that will let it fly. I will call you on it and I will tell you then and there." Of the secretary who quit her job because she could not accept Isabel in the role of chief of the section, Isabel said, "I would give her work to do, and she wouldn't do it. I would tell her something, and she would roll her eyes, and it was very disrespectful behavior. I was just not going to tolerate it, so she got a bad performance review and she left." Janet, Thalia, and Isabel's narratives all demonstrate how having high expectations was met differently, including by Latinas in supportive roles. Some were in a position to demand adherence, but others accommodated the resistance they experienced, doing work or experiencing inconvenience their male counterparts did not have to perform.

## AGE, AUTHORITY, AND COMPETENCE QUESTIONED

Latina/o doctors were cognizant of the stereotypical social identities and phenotypes that were associated with being a doctor. Many of them were explicitly made aware of the fact that they did not fit the mold of what a doctor is presumed to look like. Thomas, an internal medicine physician, described the occupation as a "white man's game and workmanship." Physicians noted that patients played a role in this practice. Vicki, a thirty-five-year-old family medicine physician, described an instance where a patient told her she did not fit the mold because she was not "white, old, and with gray hair." Not fitting the mold had negative repercussions for Latina/o doctors of both sexes, but to varying degrees, as gender intersected with age and larger cultural status beliefs about American doctors.

Both Latina/o doctors described instances where they were not readily accepted as doctors and where patients assumed they were not the attending doctor because they looked "too young." However, Latina doctors stated it was more common for patients to mistake them for someone who held a lower-status health occupation. This is in line with the Chicana/Latina lawyers in García-López and Segura's study, who subdued cultural aspects of their appearance—such as wearing their hair in a *trenza* [traditional single braid] or Virgin Mary gold chains—to avoid being misidentified and racialized as service workers.[23] Luisa, age thirty-six, explained that because of her age and gender, she was commonly mistaken for staff of a lower occupational status. "In general, people don't think I'm the doctor. They think I'm a nurse, or I'm an assistant or housekeeping, and that happens to me a lot. . . . Patients, nurses, housekeeping staff, and the OR. I had one of the housekeeping staff [ask] me if I was a doctor because I was too young and female." Numerous Latina doctors reported their family, peers, and patients thought that they were nurses, especially if they were young.[24]

Beyond dealing with the constant skepticism about being doctors, Latino/a doctors also reported that because of their relatively younger ages, nurses, patients, medical students, and other doctors would challenge their judgment or expertise. Mario, thirty-seven years old, described how his age and being Mexican contributed to patients questioning his expertise. Older patients feel "if you are a minority or you are too young, you may not have received appropriate education." Mario explained that on top of being young, patients were skeptical about his credentials because they assumed Latino doctors were not adequately trained. Rocío, who was thirty-seven years old with ten years of practice, shared a few incidents that made her believe people did not respect her and value her opinion because she was a "young woman." In one of these instances, Rocío was assigned to treat a patient who happened to be the son of a prominent person. Her colleagues undermined her by asking an older, white, male doctor about his perspective on the patient's care instead of directly speaking to her. Frustrated, she said,

> Instead of coming to me, they went straight to him! He's not even officially on the case. It's me! But he's the name everyone knows; he's more established even though I've been here five years. . . . I was the one doing the research and came up with the diagnosis and figured out the treatment plan, but still, they were going to him.

Alicia faced similar challenges but from nurses. "There's a lot of jealousy. Like 'Who are you to give me an order? You're only 28 years old and I'm 45!' There's that kind of thing going on a lot with the nurses in the workplace."

Elivet narrated an unpleasant interaction with an Asian physician:

> I was at a dinner dance [work event] with my husband and I was very made up. . . . I curled my hair, and I was wearing a nice dress. [An Asian male doctor] commented to me about being Donald Sterling's girlfriend [that is, like the much younger girlfriend of a famously racist white man in his eighties]. My husband is Mexican and very fair-skinned. . . . [My husband] took it, like saying, 'Nice job guy' [elbowing]. . . . like he was kind of congratulating my husband for getting this hot chick who could be some dumb bimbo, right? I was very offended because I was like, 'I'm the doctor here!'

The Asian doctor's assumption that Elivet's husband was a white man who held more power and prestige than her was very offensive to Elivet, a thirty-six-year-old darker-skinned Mexican woman, and it made her feel that broadcasting her femininity undermined her claim to competence.

Laura, age thirty-two, expressed how being a young family medicine doctor sometimes led to unwanted attention from patients and difficult interactions. She said,

> There have been instances where I've been hit on by patients. A lot of times I'll go in and, they're like, 'How old are you?' That's the first question I get asked. 'You must be eighteen right out of college.' That makes me feel like they don't trust me or they're not taking me seriously. So, you have to put your best foot forward and kind of not let that affect you, but it does a little.

Laura surmised her young age was an opening for unwanted attention, and even though she tried to brush it off, it still affected her confidence.

Men doctors in the sample were more likely to say they tried to overcome the ageism colleagues and patients subjected them to by "proving themselves" or subtly modifying their physical appearance. Men were more likely than women to say that despite being young, they could "prove" their competence and gain respect from patients and colleagues. Roger, a Mexican American trauma surgeon, believed the ageism he experienced from his colleagues was temporary and he merely needed to prove his capabilities to be treated as an equal. They challenged his medical knowledge to have him prove himself.

> Early on, some of the older cardiologists or pulmonologists were a little intimidated by this young Latino guy. . . . I'm not so sure that was a racial thing. I think that was a new buck in town. Thinking we need to put him in his place. I thought there was—not hazing, but there was a little bit of a period . . . the first six months I started working that I gotta prove myself.

Similarly, Esteban, thirty-eight years old, who had been in practice for nine years, described how he changed his appearance to command more respect and to put age-related questions to rest. Esteban found that growing out a beard made him look older. It also made him more masculine. "I never had a beard until I was in residency. . . . I grew it out. I kept getting that [age] question. I did have some patients who were hesitant for me to do procedures. I would have to talk them into it. And then, in the end, they're comfortable with my knowledge base." Cecilia Ridgeway notes that age intersects with high-status occupations as those perceived as older are recognized as more worthy and competent than younger individuals, like Esteban and Roger, at work.[25] In both, questions about their competence were temporary and faded over time.

Women had fewer options, as accentuating their femininity might subject them to disrespect. At sixty-two years old, Cecilia had stopped worrying about this and did "the whole shebang." She wore Chanel pink suits, high heels, nail polish, and hair dye. Getting older helped Latinas to avoid age-related stigma. While being older lessened the amount of skepticism surrounding Latina doctors' expertise, gendered and racialized stereotypes of Latinas in professional occupations meant they were still frequently mistaken for holding less prestigious health-care occupations or were taken less seriously.

## "YOU HAVE TO BE A ROBOT": MANAGING EMOTIONS

In her book *Gender Trials: Emotional Lives in Contemporary Law Firms*, Jennifer Pierce examined gender-appropriate emotional labor for trial lawyers and legal assistants.[26] She found that men lawyers perform the male-stereotyped work of aggression, winning at all costs, and humiliating coworkers. Women legal assistants, on the other hand, had to use their intuition to anticipate people's needs, reassure and provide support to coworkers, and be pleasant and lighthearted. While Latina doctors noted that they showed compassion in their communication styles with patients, Latino doctors said they were expected to be stern and serious, not unlike the trial lawyers in Pierce's research. Antonio felt this requirement did not align with his cultural norms as a Latino. He said,

> There's a stereotype of doctors. The meaner you are, the sterner you are. . . . But it seems like Latinos aren't like that. It's more flowing. It's not robotic. . . . It's very easy going and then eventually it gets to a point where you're like, 'This is what you should do but these [options] are also acceptable.'

Here, Antonio elucidates the flexibility in his self-presentation with his patients. Instead of adopting a stern demeanor, as many Latinas were encouraged to do, he was able to implement an interactive discussion with his patients, where he incorporated them into their health-making decisions.

However, along with managing their self-presentation, Latina physicians also indicated that they were encouraged to manage their emotions. Elena, who experienced blatant gendered racism from the chairman who conducted her residency interview, dealt with his comments by holding in her emotions because in her mind "crying or running off" would validate the low opinion he had of her. Joan Cassell notes that white men surgeons could throw tantrums and complain, but tensions escalated when women exhibited this behavior.[27] Elivet described a time when she was critical of her chief's leadership skills and the consequences:

> He [the chief] exploded right away. He got up and slammed his [clipboard] down. They're two older [white] men [in the room]. I did feel intimidated. At a conference, they were questioning me like, 'Why did you feel like you could talk to your chief that way? You can't be emotional that way. You have to be a robot.' Nobody wants their doctor to be a robot. But what I've noticed is, that I think if a male colleague had made some kind of comment about his leadership skills or about anything else like that, it wouldn't have exploded that way. I think it was because it was coming from a female provider, younger than him, and so he felt offended.

Elivet received a lot of negative feedback about this incident from staff, other physicians, and nurses, so she apologized. Despite her apology, she was removed from a prominent committee following the incident, a committee where Latina physicians and women of color providers, in general, are rarely present. She described this:

> He took it to the next level. He removed me from a committee that I was on as a retaliation. They refused to admit that it was a retaliation. They were like, 'We're doing it so you can concentrate on whatever.' I'm like, 'It's silly because that meeting was during my lunchtime. I wasn't taking anybody's time. I was driving there on my own time.'

Ayu Saraswati describes this dynamic as *emotion as an instrument of power*.[28] Men can freely express their emotions in public arenas without repercussions. Sofia, a 1.5-generation Guatemalan physician was convinced that gender and ethnic disparities mattered when she was spoken to "in an unprofessional manner" and when her boundaries would get overstepped or crossed more easily than white men who were well-represented in the intensive care unit (ICU). Most Latina physicians felt that they had to repress their emotions and remain stoic until they found a space where they could express them, such as with family members. Early experiences with gender bias on the job caught up to another respondent. Yvette would only cry in front of her mother. She recalled,

> [W]hen I was younger, I did cry. *'Mami porque esta persona me dijo eso?'* [Mom, why did this person tell me this?] My mom said, 'Toughen up! People are going to judge you because you are a woman or because of the color of your hair and body size, but that's their issue, not yours. ¡*Aguántate y agarrate tus huevos!'* [hold tight and grab your nuts!]

Either Yvette had taken her mother's advice, or over time she became more equipped not to mind. Now, she said, "I just let it slide. I am like whatever and that's his bias. I don't let it bother me just because I am at a different level now." Emotion management was crucial for Latina clinicians. Otherwise, they ran the risk of facing repercussions and workplace retaliation from coworkers who were higher up in the chain of command.

Medical institutions have been characterized as highly gendered and racialized organizations. Everyone in the hierarchy, from attendings and residents all the way to patients, is complicit in maintaining this inequality and status bias. Status bias in the medical profession manifests itself in different ways and those working in the "token" context often find themselves doing additional work—like interpretation—that others performing the same job are not asked to do. No matter how accomplished Latina doctors are, they face gendered racism, and their achieved high occupational status is questioned.

Performing equity work yields different types of racialized labor tasks depending on the group in question. Speaking Spanish was a professional ethnic skill that respondents, especially Latinas, saw as an asset during medical school (giving them more opportunities) but became a source of exploitation and liability for women of color physicians who moved up in the medical hierarchy. Moreover, microaggressions toward Latina doctors by nurses and staff increase such labor, as does racialized sexual harassment from patients and other doctors, something men never encountered. Latina clinicians coped by manipulating their voices and otherwise reducing their broadcast of femininity as well as emotion. Men could exhibit a range of emotions, but women had to be as controlled as possible.

The culturally competent tasks Latina physicians are expected to perform constitute a distinct burden that combines with gender exclusion and ethnic expectations to significantly overtask them. Even though both men and women physicians faced cultural taxation[29] from patients and doctors, immigrant Spanish-speaking women patients, who were more likely to seek regular health care than men, preferred Latina doctors, and therefore they bore a higher burden. Patients gravitated toward them. Bilingual and bicultural abilities primed Latinas for more uncompensated and unacknowledged work, creating a gendered cultural tax. The gendered cultural tax is a covert workload escalator, and like high blood pressure or hypertension, it can be a silent professional killer for bilingual and bicultural Latina physicians if they are not allocated support or recognized as professionals with unique strengths. The danger may be particularly high for bilingual Latinas working as tokens in otherwise all or predominantly white contexts, as they will often find themselves being over-included in tasks that others performing the same job are not asked to do or cannot do. These implicit status biases then shape people's quotidian interactions and take on systematically similar forms over multiple encounters, producing cumulative and cascading disadvantages for Latinas. Gender status beliefs are further used against high-status Latinas by co-ethnics in cross-category (nurses) and within-category (Latino doctors) interactions. Latina/o clinicians provide indispensable cultural resources for their patients, coworkers, and the medical profession as a whole, but their efforts are often invisibilized and deemed disposable, even though patients request and desperately desire them. Organizations need to invest in them to ensure that they can provide beneficial care to their patients. In the next chapter, I highlight how colorism, gender, and immigration collide in medicine, producing a range of outcomes for Latina/o clinicians. Their narratives add texture, nuance, and complexity to examinations of phenotype and minority representation in science.

# 6.

# SHADES OF RACISM

"I have benefited [from colorism] and I have been harmed by it."
—DR. ELENA ORTIZ, Ob-Gyn, Mexican American

"I am obviously very white on the outside, but very brown on the inside."
—DR. ENRIQUE CALDERON, Surgeon, Cuban

"SOMETIMES YOU CAN'T IGNORE the racism," said Soraida[1], a neurologist who self-identified as a "darker-skinned Puerto Rican," the sole Afro-Latina doctor I interviewed.[2] As a Puerto Rican, she did not experience any legal immigration challenges, and she said that although the rest of her family still lives on the island she was not a "first-generation" immigrant.[3] While her two older sisters had studied medicine on the island and practiced there, Soraida had attended a university on the US East Coast and now worked at a big hospital in metropolitan Los Angeles. She is a deep brown-complected woman with black curls that were pulled back into a low ponytail. When I asked Soraida in Spanish how she self-identified racially or ethnically, she answered in English for the first time in the interview, saying, "In Puerto Rico, I am Puerto Rican. . . . [On the US mainland] you have to decide what it is that you are." In line with others' research on Afro-Latine people in the United States, she had to choose and specify a racial identity on the mainland,[4] a concern that did not arise in Puerto Rico. She continued in English,

> Coming to the United States was a little bit of a cultural clash. In Puerto Rico you are Puerto Rican. There are white, Black, and all sorts of colors in the same family, so I have always thought of myself as Puerto Rican. I'm the darker one at my house [darker than either of her sisters], but never really thought about it until I came to the United States. Everybody seemed to point it out and ask me.

In this chapter, I show how colorism exacerbates or shields (depending on their skin tone) Latina/o physicians from assumptions about incompetence from fellow non-Latine doctors, other health personnel, and patients. Soraida experienced subtle racism from the aspiring medical students she was entrusted to train daily. She explained that white medical student trainees generally thought they were "smarter" than she was or that she "must have missed something," an evaluation she attributed both to the fact that many had attended Ivy League undergraduate schools and that based on the color of her skin, they assumed she had completed part of her training in the Caribbean. She described asserting her expertise by telling them, "I see that you're having difficulty with this concept, so I am just going to tell you the following." They seemed shocked to recognize how much she knew. "I will try to teach them nicely and carefully with detail. Sometimes they can't stop [themselves] because they have to prove that they know better." She looked down and shook her head side to side to signal her scorn.

Yet, Soraida narrated that she did not have the experiences of a Black doctor. She recognized her liminal racial position in medicine in part through the experiences of her husband. As she described, her husband is a statuesque lighter-skinned African American neck surgeon who is "assertive and very smart," a combination that didn't "go over well" in his career. Citing recent cases of police killings of unarmed Black men,[5] she emphasized the inescapable nature of racism that African Americans in the United States face; she felt that her deflection tactics reflected some degree of race privilege in some spheres. We know that skin tone biases produce cumulative advantages and disadvantages among racial groups,[6] and the education Soraida worked so hard to attain as a Puerto Rican educated in the Caribbean and Maryland schools could not protect her from racism and disrespect. I argue that for Latina/o practitioners who occupy a privileged occupational status, their achieved high social status only provides partial protection from gender and racial discrimination when compared to those who more closely embody the phenotypic demographic characteristics that medicine already privileges. Latina/o physicians recognized that their experiences with racism in the workplace were distinct from those of their racially white or Asian coworkers. Whiteness and the masculinization of the occupation are weighty organizational mainstays that determine structural outcomes and influence resource allocation in distinct ways for Latina/o bilingual men and women doctors of various hues.

In the previous chapter, I demonstrated how powerful gender status beliefs hierarchically pushed Latino men above Latinas in medicine. Here, I elucidate how Latina/o physicians of various hues move through the world and how they describe their encounters with racial discrimination in the elite, white, heteronormative organization of medicine. I incorporate gender into an intersectional analysis to deepen the conceptualization of colorism offered by scholars who examine these dynamics within Latinidad.[7] I argue that the intersection of gender, phenotype, class, nationality, and time produced a range of structural outcomes for those who are perceived to be 1) white Latinos/as; 2) those who are mestizos and note they appear racially ambiguous; and 3) those who share that they are decidedly non-ambiguously Latine. How these racial microaggressions are interpreted or explained away varied by physicians' observed race—the race others believe them to be.[8] Latino physicians who are white-presenting[9] in their appearance exhibited what scholars call a privileged marginality, where they were praised for knowing more than one language and were apportioned more resources in ways that darker-skinned men and women like Soraida, and white-presenting Latinas, were not. On the other hand, lighter-skinned mestizos whose observed race was perceived to be white were exposed to what Leslie Picca and Joe Feagin call backstage racist behaviors by their coworkers and patients.[10] Opportunity structures for those who were decidedly non-ambiguously Latine were affected by the "immigrant shadow," the notion that all Latines are poor and uneducated.

My research assistants and I did not measure skin tone; instead, physicians shared their own perceptions of how their phenotype impacted their experiences (or not) in the medical elite space. Before beginning the interview, the doctors filled out a demographic questionnaire that asked them how they self-identified racially or ethnically. Their responses varied, with many of them using national origin (for example, Puerto Rican or Colombian), hyphenated (Mexican American), pan-ethnic (Hispanic or Latina), or politicized labels (Xicano or Chicana), as Appendix A shows. The physicians interviewed were fully aware that Latines ran the gamut in phenotype from black hair and brown eyes to blond hair and blue eyes, and they recognized the vast array of hues within the Latine community and their own families. Often, Latina/o doctors themselves indicated in interviews that other people had "mistaken" them for white or that they were "lighter-skinned" compared to "darker-skinned" siblings and relatives. Many reflected on racist interactions their coworker colleagues experienced in the workplace. I coded for this as well, noting the external ascriptions of every doctor.

Latinidad encompasses a range of skin tones and ethnic markers.[11] While the doctors I spoke with reflect the heterogeneity of the Latina/o experience in terms of social location, Latina/o physicians in California in the United States do not reflect the skin color diversity of the Latina/o population broadly; physicians tend to be lighter-complected than Latinas/os generally, and among my interlocutors only Soraida identified as Afro-Latina in the US racial classification system.[12] However, some US-born or raised mestizo physicians who appeared racially ambiguous in my sample reported racial discrimination because they were exposed to backstage racist behaviors. They acknowledged the benefit of being white-presenting but did not self-identify as racially white because of racialization processes of poor Latines in the United States.[13] Complicating the issue, skin color is named and understood differently in other countries.[14] People themselves are also not reliable reporters of skin tone.[15] There are consequences of imposing monochromatic racial schemas on research participants because they may not account for the unique lived experiences of culturally shared understandings of race and color—on racial identification, stratification, and inequality.[16]

Participants' reports generally aligned with a 2021 report published by the Pew Research Center that explains that Latines in the US may face discrimination because they are Hispanic (a form of racism). Still, the degree of discrimination may vary based on skin color, with those of darker shades experiencing more incidents.[17] According to Pew, skin tone is heavily tied to discrimination experiences for Latines, with nearly 60 percent noting that having a lighter skin color helps at least a little in their ability to get ahead in the country these days. While some felt that other factors, such as education and legal status, were bigger contributors to success than skin color, most indicated that skin color can help or hurt one's life chances of getting ahead in the United States today. Their comments suggest that participants in my study agreed.

## PRIVILEGED MARGINALITY: WHITE-PRESENTING LATINOS IN WHITE

I met Antonio through my mother. I had driven her to the new podiatrist's[18] office that her medical insurance provider sent her to and sat in the waiting room because of COVID-19 protocols, contemplating the Asian American office assistant and worrying that my mother would need an interpreter. When she emerged and said, *"El doctor es Latino y le pregunté si lo podías entrevistar para tú libro"* [The doctor is Latino and I asked him if you could interview him for your book], I was very surprised. Antonio had ocean blue eyes as well as pepper gray hair; neither my mother nor I would have realized he was Latino if not for the fact that he addressed her in Spanish. My mother was ecstatic that she was able to help me recruit a Latino physician. She reported that they were able to talk about her life back in her village in Santa Juana, Zacatecas, in Mexico. For my part I was pleased that she finally had a doctor with whom she could communicate her ailments without needing me in the room, a topic I discuss in greater detail in the next chapter.[19]

I interviewed Antonio a couple of days later in his office with our masks on, sitting further than six feet away from him. His office was decorated with pictures of his family and his children at their sporting events. Various medals from the half and full marathons that Antonio ran were also on display. He filled out the demographic questionnaire, indicating that his father was born in Ecuador and his mother was born in New Hampshire. Antonio was multiracial, white, and Ecuadorian, and was born and raised in Los Angeles. While Antonio felt that he was mistaken for a resident or an attending "all the time" when he was in medical school, before his hair grayed, he explained that he never noticed any racial discrimination toward him in his medical office because he did not "look the part." Through his slight accent, he elaborated, "Race hasn't affected me. In my case, it doesn't. . . . It's probably helped me because I'm able to go either way. At first, *they see me,* they [other Latinos] don't think I speak Spanish or understand that aspect."

White-presenting Latino physicians—doctors whose observed race was white but did not self-identify that way socially—rarely reported exclusion or marginalization from other physicians or patients in medicine. This was especially the case for white-presenting Latino physicians who worked in locations with large Spanish-speaking immigrant populations in Southern California. Patients and coworkers were surprised to discover they were bilingual and praised them for it, while darker-skinned Latinas/os generally encountered an assumption that they were (or should be) bilingual. This resulted in receiving more patient referrals, and white-presenting physicians were also provided with the means to sustain themselves (additional interpreters or resources) in ways that darker-skinned physicians were not.

When I asked Antonio if he had experienced any prejudice or discrimination in the workplace, he responded that he did not think so. "If I have, I haven't noticed it. I usually attribute it to other things if it was." When I asked him what other things, he said "personality." He explained,

> Race is kind of interesting growing up here [in Los Angeles]. It never really felt like it was ever an issue because I was always kind of the minority being the light-skinned one. . . . I consider myself Hispanic because I grew up in the Spanish culture. I play soccer and grew up in LA. If I wanted to play [soccer] I had to speak Spanish to get the ball. I will joke about that because I felt like I was good enough, but they [other Latino players] don't trust you. My high school team used to make fun of me because I was one of the few, you know, light-skinned guys on the team . . . including the referees. So, I get [sic] a lot of whistles trying to get me off the field, but that's okay. Once you get past that they were always nice to you. I'm used to that.

Because Antonio was born and raised in Los Angeles, he was adept at navigating and breaking through these in-group boundaries within the Latine community. Speaking Spanish helped him. Antonio was aware of his racial privilege as a white Latino in US racial hierarchies, and he took extra measures to demonstrate this to darker-skinned co-ethnics by engaging in silly banter with them. Yet he was not above enjoying the surprise of immigrant Latine patients who assumed he could not speak Spanish and were highly impressed to learn he could. He would first engage them in English and then amaze them with his linguistic capital, a surprise they always welcomed. "I guess I kind of have the best of both worlds," he chuckled. He emphasized his respect for his immigrant patients, whom he characterized as "hard workers," and how glad he was that he could engage them with cultural competence in ways that improved patient care.

It took some time for Antonio to grow the Latine part of his practice. As a podiatrist, he primarily saw patients through referral, and other physicians did not realize when his office was new that he spoke Spanish. However, feedback from some patients had spread the word, and by the time we spoke—after six years on the job—half of his patients were Latine. In many ways, Antonio's experience reflects what sociologist Wendy Roth calls *observed race*—the race others ascribe to people.[20] He was treated as white by observers, who following interpersonal interactions changed their assessment. Like Antonio, other physicians who were mistaken for white or "looked white" reported that when they spoke Spanish people would ask them about their ethnicity and then classify them as Latine if they affirmed this background, which led to particular social outcomes, such as positive appraisals on the job. Non-white-presenting Latina/o physicians were not regarded as warmly.

With his fair skin and green eyes, Jacob's experiences were much like Antonio's. Jacob, too, spoke joyfully of seeing his Latine immigrant patients' faces light up when they realized he could communicate with them in the Los Angeles hospital where he worked. He was also conscious of phenotypical diversity among Latines because his two younger twin sisters—also adopted from Colombia—were darker in complexion and had different experiences in America than he did.

Different Latine subgroups experience US racial hierarchies in divergent ways. While South American migrant professionals can achieve relative socioeconomic success in the United States, stereotypes about South Americans abound in the United States, such as the notions that they uniformly enjoy class privilege, are white, and are "new" migrants.[21] According to sociologist Lina Rincón, South Americans are relatively successful economically in comparison to other Latina/o/e national-origin groups. However, her study of information technology professionals suggest that South Americans experience a *privileged marginality* due to their racialization and unstable legal status.[22] Researchers often use middle-class descriptors to describe Colombians, such as that they are "entrepreneurs," "well-educated," and speak "good Spanish."[23] The white Colombians in Rincón's research do not encounter marginalization due to their physical features because most are light-skinned and, unlike Mexicans and Central Americans do not experience criminalization. Jacob and Antonio seem to share these advantages, and unlike Colombian migrants in the IT sector, they did not confront workplace marginalization and stigmatization because of their ethnic affiliation and accents.[24] Both were trained and educated in American schools and possessed citizenship status, which also protected them from the anxiety about legal status that was common among those Rincón studied. The general understanding that their Spanish language skills were extremely valuable in their jobs seemed to confer an advantage unattached to any disadvantage.

Arnoldo was also white-presenting, although his slightly accented English sometimes raised questions. He was born in Mexico City and his family migrated to the United States when he was thirteen. From eighth to twelfth grade he lived in Miami, and then his family moved back to Mexico City, where he completed his college education in medicine before attending Harvard to receive more medical graduate training. Arnoldo explained that he enjoyed living in Miami because there was a predominance of Spanish there. But he said that many people took him for a "Mexican Jew" at Harvard and he never felt out of place there. It seemed that he fit the mold of what a scientist looks like. His accent often garnered him praise and respect from his coworkers and patients. Most of Arnoldo's patients were racial/ethnic minorities and working class and he spoke to them in Spanish. While women doctors described pleading for Spanish-speaking personnel, as we saw in the previous chapter, Arnoldo was assigned a nurse and another staff person who would help him throughout his workday. Skin color is an important factor for within-group resource heterogeneity, and here we see that skin color (and gender) matter in allocating additional staff or resources to doctors.

Arnoldo's feelings about his privilege were complex. He explained that he felt "guilty" because he did not experience the exclusion that many Latine students face in schools today and that "he missed out" on racism. While he realized that Latines faced exclusion because of Donald Trump's anti-immigration and anti-Latino rhetoric, Arnoldo made attempts to understand US racial hierarchies. He even attended White People 4 Black Lives Matter (WP4BL) dialogues to learn more.

To summarize: white-presenting Latino physicians reaped the rewards of white racial privilege in the US racial structure, and their Spanish-speaking abilities, even with accented English, were an advantage in elite medical spaces.

## White-Presenting Latina Physicians

Skin tone mattered significantly in medical interactions regardless of ethnicity, national origin, or USMG/IMG status. Jazmín, who was Colombian and an IMG, and Lizet, who was a USMG and daughter of working-class Mexican immigrants, also presented as light-skinned and white-presenting, and both acknowledged that they experienced little racial discrimination at work because stereotypes and controlling images of Latinas as deviant or hyperfertile[25] were not projected onto them. Jazmín had experience working both in Beverly Hills and a county hospital in LA, and she remarked, "I don't think people know that I'm Latina, so I don't think that I'm targeted or looked at differently." Upon further reflection, she specified that her experiences were also influenced by the fact that she came to the United States when she was around thirty years old to work at UCLA as an elite immigrant on a fellowship:

> With this huge accent coming from Colombia, people have been very accepting. I don't feel . . . it has been a lot of work for me in my transition. I worked hard to be where I am today, but I [would] have to work more if I was from here. I have to prove myself but overall, this country has been very open to me.

Lizet also explained that she had a very slight accent indicative of a native Spanish speaker that sometimes gave her away as something other than white, but because of her blond hair, most people assumed she was a white woman even though she was the daughter of Mexican immigrants.

Raquel's experience suggests that fair-skinned women faced a more complex opportunity structure than their male counterparts. The US-born child of Mexican immigrants, she was fair-skinned with pink undertones and a wiry blond bob. When I asked if she had ever experienced racism or discrimination, Raquel answered,

> Never. And I think part of it is because I'm not dark-skinned. My colleague, who's dark-skinned? Yes, I've heard Caucasian patients say they don't want to see him because they felt his English wasn't that good and they'll make excuses like that. The first thing patients say is, 'Oh I couldn't understand his English.'

Raquel felt that her fairer skin protected her from racist patients who would mistake her for a white woman, something that her darker-skinned coworkers could not escape, especially when they spoke with an accent. She noted that she was more likely to experience racist microaggressions outside of the medical workplace and in the suburban neighborhood where she resided with her Chinese American radiologist husband. One door-to-door salesman asked for the homeowner; when she answered the door, they thought she was the maid.

At the same time, Raquel could speak Spanish, and like other Latinas, but unlike Antonio, Jacob, or Arnoldo, she received additional work duties with no additional support. Unlike white-presenting Latino physicians who were praised for speaking Spanish and were apportioned resources, white-presenting Latinas were rarely lauded by their coworkers.

## BACKSTAGE RACISM ENCOUNTERED BY
## LIGHT-SKINNED *DOCTORES*

Presenting as white, and not self-identifying that way, meant being exposed to coworkers' *backstage racist behaviors*—racial attitudes and behaviors that whites exhibit when they believe no one who is not white is present.[26] Several white-presenting Latina/o doctors acknowledged their phenotypic privilege but also felt that it came with harms, especially when they were privy to racist remarks from their coworkers who thought that because of their phenotype, they upheld white supremacist ideologies. This was the case for those who were raised working-class and the US-born children of immigrants more so than those who were foreign-born and arrived in the United States as older, highly skilled professionals. Socioeconomic class status mattered in these perceptions. Because USMG lighter-skinned physicians were mostly raised in poorer families where there was a spectrum of phenotypes or were in close contact with families and communities that were discriminated against for being Latine, they also felt personally wounded and hurt by comments that were not directly targeted toward them.

Pedro, a 1.5-generation Mexican immigrant, explained that he had never "been discriminated against as a male" and chortled when he said he looked white. "It's funny how that plays out because if people don't know my name, they assume that I'm [white]. People are more liberal to say comments and then I'm like, 'That was stereotypical or racist.'" Pedro noted that he would get frustrated by some of the racist comments his colleagues would make about uninsured Latine immigrant patients. He acknowledged that he tried to find a balance between being an advocate for his patients but tried not to socially distance himself from his colleagues.

Camelia, who was in her third year in medical school, said, "Sometimes I have like a privilege because I'm a lighter-skinned Mexican. A lot of people don't think I'm a minority." The anti-Latine sentiment she described was similar to what Pedro experienced:

> As you can see, I'm like a lighter-skinned Latina. A lot of times people don't even realize I am Mexican. They act very surprised when I tell them that I speak Spanish. One of the supervisors just the other day was like, 'We're gonna go see this patient.' I say, 'I already saw them.' He says, 'Well they're only Spanish-speaking.' I say, 'Yeah, I speak Spanish.' He looked back at me and literally looked at me up and down, surprised that I had said that. He kept walking and once we were in the room I was able to translate everything because I'm a fluent Spanish speaker, my first language.

Camelia perceived a racist subtext to her colleague's confusion. She clarified:

> He acted very surprised that I was Mexican and that I spoke Spanish that well, which bothers me in a lot of ways because people always say, 'Oh, you don't look Mexican.' What does looking Mexican mean? Mexico has such a wide range of people because we come from so many different backgrounds. You can't say you don't look Mexican. That's the only little microaggression that I've had. . . . There have been other instances, but this is the one that has stood out to me the most because this was very blunt.[27]

For both Camelia and Pedro, being the children of working-class Mexican immigrants influenced how they interpreted racist microaggressions toward them and their co-ethnic community.

Light-skinned Mexican mestizo physicians were not always pro-tected from prejudice. Luisa recalled a woman patient who said she didn't want a woman physician once she saw her walk into the room. Luisa was convinced that the woman actually "did not want a Mexican doctor." Luisa was philosophical; she said, "That's fine and she got to see my white male colleague."

These microaggressions were also experienced by light-skinned Latina/o physicians who were not of Mexican heritage. Perla was largely concerned with misapprehensions about the status of Puerto Rico, where she was born, although her family moved to Irvine, CA, when she was one month old. Perla described herself as "100 percent Puerto Rican."[28] Her coworkers often made remarks indicating they thought that Puerto Rico was a foreign country in Latin America. She also experienced derogatory comments about Puerto Ricans while she was giving patients care. "Sometimes patients would talk about [Don-ald] Trump [when he was president from 2017–2021] throwing us paper towels or giving us dog treats. Treating us like animals." She recalled that once she had accidentally enclosed her birth certificate in a medi-cal textbook that she sold online on Amazon. While the recipient was courteous enough to mail the document back to her, the accompany-ing note said, "I'm returning this to someone who was not born in the United States," a line Perla interpreted as questioning her right to US citizenship. Skin tone only provided high status and light-skinned Lati-nas/os fleeting protection from backstage racism.

## "ANYTHING BUT MEXICAN": RACIALIZATION IN SCIENCE

Light-skinned mestiza/o physicians, especially those who were of Mex-ican origins and were born or came of age in the US, narrated that self-identifying as Mexican was met with racial stigma and disdain in medi-cine by their colleagues. Rudy Acuña's groundbreaking book *Anything But Mexican: Chicanos in Contemporary Los Angeles* chronicles how working-class Mexican Americans in Los Angeles were blamed for the decline of the city.[29] I use his title in the subheading to explicate how Latina/o doctors felt that they were racialized as incapable of achieving success and less intelligent in science-related orbits. Elena, whose skin was a light golden brown, hesitated to talk to me about the impact of racism and colorism in her life. "I haven't thought about it in a long time," she said. My questions prompted Elena to reflect on her experience over a lifetime in STEM. She told me, "I have benefited [from colorism] and I have been harmed by it. Can you look at me and figure it out?"—meaning, could I decipher her ethnicity just from looking at her? Elena identified as Chicana and was born in Pleasanton, California, a suburb in the Bay Area where most residents were Asian or white. "Guess what people say and project onto me?" she prodded. I remained mum but smiled, and hoped she would answer her question. She did.

Elena explained that she had self-identified with the politicized ethnic label Chicana "more in undergrad" and now at this point in her life and in her career thought of herself as Mexican American. She felt that "race became less of a problem" as she moved up the higher echelons of the educational hierarchy and into medicine, in ways similar to the Black doctors in Adia Wingfield's work who noted racism an aberration.[30] Elena felt as if she was "less Mexican" as an undergraduate at a prominent University of California campus because she wasn't "dark enough," but this feeling got "better over time" as she took ethnic studies courses and learned more about her roots and the social conditions that Mexicans living in the United States faced.

Things changed in medical school. "There was no time for that [to think about race or ethnicity]," Elena said. She experienced racial injury, but she would try and brush it off. "You can't cry and run off [in medical school]." However, Elena felt that the higher she went in her career the more there was "no [racism] problem there. Never felt it." She felt that people's difficulty determining her ethnicity played a role, especially now that her hair had lost its natural tint to gray. She told me that people often asked her, "Where did you learn to speak Spanish?" or "Are you South American?" They usually guessed she was from Spain, Iran, or Italy, but never Mexico. Given that Mexicans are the largest immigrant group in California, this is striking. Elena surmised that people assessed her as anything but Mexican because they assumed that Mexicans were incapable of becoming doctors.

Rocío, who was a third-generation Mexican American, reported a similar experience. Of her phenotype and its effect in the medical workplace she said, "I'm pretty pale and people will ask me all the time 'What are you?' And when I say Mexican, they seem somewhat disappointed. They're like, 'We thought you'd be a mix of South American.' I'm like, 'just Mexican.'" She was, she reported, "not as white" as her younger brother. Interestingly, despite being a later-generation Mexican American and lighter-skinned, Rocío still felt that self-identifying as Mexican was met with scorn, mainly in relation to Asians in medicine who, Lata Murti notes, are perceived to be superior healers.[31] Scholars have detailed how Asian Americans and Latines are academically profiled in majority-minority schools, with positive appraisals attributed to Asians in relation to Mexicans.[32] This extended to medicine as well.

Rocío explained her general perception that Asians and Asian Americans had a greater advantage in the medical field compared to Latina/os thus:

> In medicine what's considered an underrepresented minority is not the same as in life. Asian Americans, South [Asians], and East Asian Americans are overrepresented in medicine. There are a lot of Chinese doctors and there are a lot of Indian doctors. Although they are a minority in America, in medicine they are not.

Because South Asians and East Asians have higher representations in medicine, Rocío described that discrimination took a different form for

Latinas/os in this elite space. Because it was more common to see Asians wear the white coat, their presence or intelligence wasn't questioned in the ways that that Latinas/os had to prove their competence. Rather, while Asians experience racial discrimination in other realms, Rocío insinuated that the model minority status allotted seemingly positive stereotypes not accorded to Latina/o doctors.[33] Asians do have the highest educational attainment, highest median income, and lowest unemployment rate of any racial or ethnic group in the United States,[34] and tend to enter STEM-related careers.[35] Research also shows that they are the racial group with the most socioeconomic gap between ethnic groups in the US.[36] Moreover, Asian men are 112 percent more likely to be executives or hold leadership positions than Asian women. Asian American women are also the subgroup who are affected by racial discrimination in both their personal and professional lives and are the least likely to ascend to positions of power when compared with Asian men and white women.[37] However, South Asians are more likely than East Asians to achieve executive leadership in the United States.[38] Some call this phenomenon the bamboo ceiling—the invisible barriers that prevent well-qualified Asian American women and men from attaining leadership positions.[39]

Latina/o doctors observed that Asian American physicians played into the model minority stereotype to their disadvantage. Raquel described an experience of discrimination by the Asian-American chief of her department. When she joined the department, he had said, "You're the first one [meaning the first Latine in the department]. I don't know what to expect from you." Most of Raquel's colleagues, including the chief, were Asian immigrants and Asian Americans and she sensed that they upheld the model minority myth of Asian excellence and intelligence by putting her down. "I don't think other people get that [kind of treatment] when they're Asian or Indian." Raquel also noticed that Asian physicians had strong social capital networks in medicine and were able to support each other because of their higher numbers in the field compared to Latines.[40]

Roger Morales, who self-identified as Chicano and was now in an administrative position, made similar observations. Like Elena, he felt that he had achieved a high occupational status within medicine that protected him from prejudice. Nonetheless, he recalled,

> I always felt that there was racial bias. . . . Sometimes when the physician was white or Asian, I feel like they were caring more [about their ideas] than mine even though I had a better grasp of the situation. . . . I haven't experienced that as an attending [at a new hospital] and especially not as a surgeon. [As] a surgeon you're the end of the line. . . . I'm in a different position now but before this, I felt it. . . . If I was Caucasian or Asian, a more traditionally accepted race in medicine, they wouldn't question you that much.

Attendings are at the top of the medical hierarchy, and as a surgeon, Roger would be the last person to see the patient. Being at the top of the hierarchy served as a protection from racial microaggressions from coworkers for Roger because it minimized his interactions with his coworkers.

Lisa, a Salvadoran with sienna-toned skin, explained that on two separate occasions the Caucasian patients that she was treating had requested an Asian doctor over her, claiming that she spoke English with a slight accent. She recalled,

> There was an intern who was Asian and had seen this patient. The interns [second years] are the ones that do a lot of the paper, a lot of the stuff, and I supervise them. I understand it was race because . . . I come in later and I know everything about everyone because [I'm the senior resident]. I am talking in English, and the patient is like, 'I don't understand you. Bring back the Asian doctor.' 'Sir, I am speaking English,' I said. He says, 'No, but I don't understand *your* English.'

Here, Lisa explained that a patient preferred an Asian-heritage intern over her because they were imagined as being a more natural fit in medicine despite her seniority.

## "DON'T YOU KNOW WHAT YOUR COWORKERS LOOK LIKE?": THE IMMIGRANT SHADOW

Men and women physicians who self-reported that they were brown mestizos/as and of working-class roots indicated that they experienced a series of racial microaggressions directed at their Latine identity. These were doctors whose melanin varied: their skin had different shades of brown and ranged from olive to deep brown tones. What they described reflected what immigration scholars call the immigrant shadow—assumptions that they have low levels of education, lack documentation, and hold low-wage and low-status jobs.

Julio, who was the child of undocumented Nicaraguan immigrants, counted off on his fingers the number of times that he encountered subtle acts of racial discrimination:

> In medical school at UCSF, while I was studying in the library, I was mistaken for a janitor. . . . There's nothing wrong with being a janitor. It's just like out of everyone there, you picked the one Latino dude to ask for the keys to unlock the janitor closet and there was an employee there. I'm like, 'Don't you know what your coworkers look like?' Come on! That was one.

Another time, Julio shared, "I was just walking down the stairs, coming out of the medical building [at UCSF] and some random [person] was like, 'Oh, your name's Jesús?' So, for me, it's like there are so few Latinos at UCSF that this white lady saw a Latino face, and was like, 'That must be Jesús.' And there are thousands of people there [on campus]." Exasperated, recalling this, Julio cried out, "Jesus Christ!" That was two.

Coworkers also compounded the problem. Julio's white doctor colleagues who worked at a hospital in the Bay Area, had witnessed him being mistaken for a construction worker in the cafeteria, and they would needle him about it. Julio described, "They were like 'Are you a construction worker?' 'No,' I responded. 'Oh, but you look like a construction worker,' they continued. [My coworker] was like, 'Doesn't he look like a construction worker?' [pointing at Julio] It was maddening. I guess embarrassing. I was angrier than anything else. I was just like, 'you're an asshole,' type of deal. That was another one. They just wouldn't let it go." This scenario in which white coworkers used racist humor in the workplace aligned with others' research on people of color in predominantly white professional spaces.[41] This was three.

Much like Black male nurses who experience challenges in white-dominated spaces,[42] Julio struggled with the fact that he didn't automatically get the respect that he thought he should. "If I was a white man [I'd] get it right away." When I asked Julio how his Latine patients referred to him, he said "Doctor. Always! The only patients that call me by my first name are white Americans." Julio was careful to always wear his white coat. He even wore it when patients would not be able to see it behind closed doors. "You just see my face [in certain circumstances]. [But the coat is] still like a barrier. It's still like fighting to be seen." He went on,

> As an attending physician, I always make sure that I have my badge on, or I always wear my white coat. I do it on purpose. Some of my colleagues don't. They don't have a reason but the reason I do it is . . . one time . . . I was a medical student, and a little boy was walking down the hallway. He was staring at me, and he whispered to his mom in Spanish, *Mami, el es doctor y es Latino,* and I was like, 'Oh my God, that was so powerful.' I felt so filled with gratitude. It was the first time he'd ever seen a Latino doctor. Because of that, I do it on purpose. So that there's no mistake that I'm a doctor.

Alejandro, on the other hand, opted not to wear his white coat on the job "most of the time" because it "didn't protect him from racism at all." He had shaved his thick black handlebar-shaped mustache and beard in medical school to appear more "professional," but felt he no longer had to manage his self-presentation because the immigrant shadow would be lurking whether he wore it or not.

Karen, in family medicine, also had mixed results in using a prop—in her case, a stethoscope—to avoid the immigrant shadow. A brown mestiza, she is the child of Mexican immigrants. Karen said,

When I was in residency people thought I was doing maintenance because the maintenance workers wore the same type of color scrubs as we doctors did. Here the nurses, doctors, and surgeons wear different colors. You can tell who is who. I used to carry my stethoscope in my pocket or belt. Twice I got asked to clean after a patient vomits by another doctor and another by a nurse. It happens [laughs] when you look at me. If I am Mexican and I am there I am probably there to clean [rather] than be a doctor.

While lighter-skinned and white-presenting Latina physicians rarely confronted controlling images[43]—hegemonic racial ideologies that permeate social institutions—of Latinas directly, brown mestizas encountered these racist incidents regularly. Ana, who was born in Santa Ana, California, talked about an incident where a male patient asked her "Were you born here?," signaling to her that he thought she lacked citizenship status.

Like Julio, Alicia, a Mexican American woman in internal medicine, experienced racist treatment from white physician friends. A white physician friend said to her once, "Well, you know, the reason why you're making it in Pasadena is, number one, you're light, you're attractive, and you don't look like a *chola* [gang member]." Alicia said, "It might have been said in a very lighthearted way, but that is discrimination. And it is in full force. . . . I always had great comebacks because the doctor [her friend] said in the next sentence, 'So, proud of you,' as he announced this in a meeting. I said, 'I am so proud of you, too. You graduated from medical school. Good job!'" She gestured as if she were patting him on the head to signal that they were both on the same level. A bright copper-toned Latina, Alicia was gregarious and dedicated to addressing and dismantling racism. She organized fundraising banquet events that would defray the costs of Latines who wanted to pursue postbaccalaureate programs. I attended the Annual Postbacc Fundraiser Program she hosted which was held at a popular Mexican restaurant in Pasadena, California, and met several doctors of color. This strategy of engaging in leadership endeavors was a form of resistance toward racist controlling images.[44]

Physician specialty also mattered for non-white-presenting male physicians, especially those who pursued fields in surgery. The child of Peruvian immigrants who settled in the San Francisco area, Samuel was careful not to reveal details that his white coworkers might read and identify with him, concerned that it might affect his relationships with them and future vertical mobility. He was reacting to a bitter experience: "I don't want to get into the details of that [racism] but there's always like bullying behavior. It was a small component of my training. I did not get treated with respect." He was the only Latino specializing in surgery at a private highly competitive university located in Northern California.

Lorenzo also felt that being a surgeon had increased his vulnerability to microaggressions. His patient coordinator had told him that patients regularly asked about his nationality.

> My patient coordinator has been asked, 'Where is he from?' She, messing with them will say, 'Well, he was born in Chicago.' They're like, 'No, where is he from?' She's like, 'He was raised in LA and went to UCLA.' 'But Contreras, where is he from? Oh, where are his parents from?' They're trying to see if I'm Mexican. I don't know if that's [because] some people might think that's a bad thing. That I'm Mexican and maybe I'm from affirmative action or not as well-qualified.

In her study of the Mexican-origin middle class, sociologist Jody Agius Vallejo examines how poverty and middle-class privilege intersect with race/ethnicity to heighten or minimize subtle racism.[45] She notes that pejorative stereotypes followed upwardly mobile Mexican Americans despite their professional accomplishments. Julio, Alejandro, and Samuel were the children of Nicaraguan, Mexican, and Peruvian immigrants, respectively, and all of these men encountered subtle forms of racism at work. Latinas/os of various ethnicities who see themselves as brown mestizos and grew up working-class in America interpret these slights as discriminatory practices.

Unlike white-passing Latino physicians who were praised for speaking Spanish, light-skinned mestizo/a Mexican and Central American physicians were rarely praised for being bilingual. Women physicians who performed this labor were simultaneously punished by their doctor coworkers and some non-Latine patients for doing so.

## COLORISM AND LANGUAGE

Brown mestizo men were regularly questioned about their expertise, educational credentials, and intelligence in their specialties in ways that their white-presenting Latino counterparts were not. Most Latina doctors also faced such questions, especially if they could not pass as white and/or spoke with a discernible accent in English. Latinas who were white-presenting, foreign-born, and spoke with an accent relayed that these questions would go away over a certain period of time after they got to know their coworkers. Elsa indicated that she "could see doubts in the eyes of the doctors" who wondered if the training she received in her hometown of Colombia was going to be as competent as theirs. With shoulder-length sleek brown gossamer hair that framed her pale white skin, she could pass as white. As she increasingly established herself in the US, she felt the questions had dissipated. Elsa recounted, "A few years ago when they didn't know me, I saw more that the interrogations were about if I was good enough but not anymore. Sometimes . . . in meetings, they'll be like, 'Oh, Latino? Okay,' because there are not that many primary investigators that are Latinos here." Elsa commented that because of her accent some of her newer patients would opt to see another doctor. Isabel Pinedo, a Brazilian fawn-brown-toned mestiza who specialized in radiology and was an IMG trained in Brazil, reported similar experiences. She said, "I know there are issues of . . . competence in looking down [on you] because you're of brown skin . . . because you speak with an accent."

Pew Research Center's survey suggests that Latina/o adults often experience being treated as if they were not smart. Forty-two percent of Latinos with darker skin indicated this happened to them, as did 34 percent of Latinos with lighter skin. Moreover, Latinos who were Spanish/English bilingual were more likely to say they had been treated this way (41 percent) than those who were dominant Spanish speakers (32 percent) and those who were dominant English speakers (29 percent).[46] Pablo, a bilingual doctor who described himself as "a shade of brown" and was the US-born son of Mexican immigrants, aligned with the Pew report. He said, "You do deal with some non-Latine patients that look at you and give a hesitant look when you say you are the physician taking care of their kid. You see that. I specifically can't say a blatant kind of racist. . . . You tend to see a lot more of the unspoken [kind]." As a brown Mexican man, Pablo was attuned to the more subtle forms of racism he felt from some non-Latine patients, as did most 1.5- and second-generation male doctors.

Miguel, a taupe brown-toned mixed Mexican and Filipino surgeon, worked with a white-appearing Latino business partner, and their differing experiences were also reflected in the Pew report. Miguel stated,

> I don't know if it's racially motivated or if some people just look [at] the color of your skin. My partner, Dr. Rivera, you might think he's Anglo. He's a light complexion, he speaks perfect English, and he speaks Spanish just as well or better. . . . I don't think he's ever been discriminated against because you look at him and it doesn't look right. You look at me? I'm dark and there's a difference if you're in a white society so to speak.

In both cases, Pablo and Miguel felt that skin tone in conjunction with the Spanish language was a source of stigma in their jobs.

Similarly, Mauricio, a tawny brown-toned Mexican physician who worked in Santa Clara in the Bay Area, explained that higher- and upper-class patients questioned him in a way that immigrant and marginalized patients never did:

I did deal with more patients and families that [were] higher, upper class. A lot of times they would ask you questions like, 'Where did you do your training? Or where'd you go to med school?' Questions that you wouldn't get at a county hospital. You could tell. People would tell you, 'My son is a VIP at Google.' I didn't care about that. There are some prejudices. . . . I can tell they were asking for a reason.

Mauricio was unhappy working for this facility and ended up doing his fellowship in an underserved community where he felt he received more trust from his Latine patients. Many of his Caucasian patients asked about his credentials before deciding whether they wanted to receive care from him. He disclosed:

I don't know if that has to do with them being affluent or if that's something they're accustomed to doing with every one of their doctors because maybe they're college-educated? . . . I worked in a clinic in Pasadena for USC. . . . Most of my patient population was affluent, professional, and Caucasian. I saw a lot of lawyers; other doctors were my patients and were professors at the college. The not-uncommon questions were, 'Where did you go to medical school? When did you graduate? How long have you been a doctor?' or, 'I looked you up and I know what your résumé is.'

Mauricio explained that white patients would look up his qualifications ahead of time and still asked questions about his credentials when they saw him in person. The privilege the white coat bestows is fleeting.

Karen, too, explained that white patients in Los Angeles County were more "critical" of her. With brown terra-cotta skin and coarse bouncy curls, she was not white-presenting. Karen revealed, "The power of what you say may not be as great as you would hope. They [white patients] are a little bit more demanding. A lot of them have some educational background and know a little bit. Most of them have access to the internet." While Karen hoped the white coat would legitimize the medical knowledge she was imparting to her white patients, its power was diluted for her in these interactions.

Similarly, Esteban, whose skin tone was a light yellow-brown, said that he received these types of questions from the white patients who he treated in the very affluent Orange County in Southern California. They wondered if he, as a Mexican-origin physician, had received his training in a foreign country.

> Early on, here in Orange County, is where—I did feel a little bit [sighs] more scrutinized. . . . It's been so many years. I felt there was some [racial] undercurrent in some of the questions I would get. 'Where you from?' Or like, 'Did you train in the US?' Things like that. 'I don't know . . . if your training is good enough.' The tone, and the way the questions were asked. I felt that here in Orange County.

This experience of having his patients probe where he received his training and questioning his citizenship status seemed particularly egregious in Orange County, because Esteban was more familiar with its more diverse and left-leaning political areas.

In the US medical profession, the conflation of race and color, while related terms, can obfuscate intra-racial stratification and inequality across contexts.[47] This chapter shows how gender intersects with phenotype and matters for stratification in medicine because it produces distinct status hierarchies and an uneven apportioning of resources for Latina/o medics. The US's Black/white binary schema contrasts with the fluid and nuanced racial categorization of Latin America, which affects how Latinos living in the US perceive their own racial identity,[48] but respondents' words reflect that ascribed characteristics such as skin tone trump achieved high-status medical degrees. Immigrant Latines, especially women and those who are darker-skinned, suffer in the process of adapting because there is a perception in the US that you can only be white or non-white.[49] Elite and foreign-born Latinas/os feel compelled to choose what they are even if they might self-identify differently in their Latin American country of origin. Quickly, if painfully, Latine migrants learn that in the US you are either white or not.

In Latin America class status tends to trump "color"; thus, a well-edu-cated, well-dressed darker-skinned person can avoid discrimination based on color or race. To be sure, colorism is present in Latin Ameri-can countries and cultures (and globally), but the white racial category is not always the reference point.[50] That is not the case in American medicine, as the doctors in this chapter came to learn.

White-presenting Latino doctors in white experience rewards and praise akin to the white men who dominate medicine. Their accents did not cause them exclusion. Rather, for them, exhibiting Spanish/English linguistic capital was a bonus to their qualifications at work because multilingual doctors are desperately needed in the job. In some ways, the privileged marginality white-presenting Latino doc-tors experience produces a glass escalator[51] effect—structural advan-tages in resource allocation versus consequences. This glass escalator effect does not extend to lighter-skinned mestizos/as in medicine who are exposed to their coworkers' and patients' backstage racist behav-iors when their observed race is perceived to be white and when they appear racially ambiguous. This was an added emotional weight that they carried, too. While their observed race was white, they did not fully resonate with nor wholly experience that form of racial privilege with their families or at work.

For Latinos/as who described themselves as unambiguously Latine, Spanish became a stigmatizing marker, and they encountered discrim-ination when they used it on the job among coworkers. Some Latinos/as described being perceived as white or Black until they spoke Span-ish, at which point their accent or use of the language led observers to reclassify them as Latine, leading to specific outcomes. Moreover, Mexican and Central American physicians who were born or came of age in the United States were exposed to US racial hierarchies in their childhoods in their families of origin and interpreted instances of dis-crimination differently than most foreign-born Latinos. Unlike white-presenting Latino physicians who were praised for speaking Spanish and received hidden advantages, light-skinned mestizo/a Mexican and Central American physicians were rarely praised for being bilingual, especially women. They faced an immigrant shadow, where they were stereotyped as poor and uneducated, and sometimes felt that there was a stigma when they revealed their ethnic identity to coworkers and staff. In these cases, the high occupational status the white coat usually confers was fleeting, as they did not experience all of its benefits.

In the next chapter, I take the reader into examination rooms to delve deeper into doctor-patient interactions and foreground the patients that clinicians care for daily to elucidate how they blend biomedical science with their patients' sociocultural realities under the crushing weight of a profit-driven medical industry that requires all health-care organizations to provide language concordant care.

# 7.

# CLINICIANS AND PATIENTS

*"La doctora que tengo me atiende. . . . Le digo a mi mujer, 'ya me va a ver la doctora.' No es por hablar mal de mi doctor [de cabecera], pero no lo podía ver por cuatro meses. A mi edad necesito que me atienda más seguido. No me atendía. Me iba a Tijuana. Allá tengo amigos que son doctores. Es rápido. ¿Por qué voy a pagar allá si tengo mi seguro? Está uno bien a gusto [aquí]."*

[The Latina doctor I have attends to me. I tell my wife, 'The doctor will see me now.' It is not to talk bad about my primary doctor, but I couldn't see him for four months. At my age, I need someone that can attend to me more frequently. He wouldn't see me. I would go to Tijuana. Some of my friends are doctors there. It's fast. But why am I going to pay over there if I have insurance? I am at ease here.]

—Cipriano

THE CO-ETHNIC DOCTOR CIPRIANO referenced is Perla, a bilingual Puerto Rican heritage physician who specializes in family medicine. Of all the Latina physicians I interviewed, Perla was one of three who had a private practice. When she wore the white coat, patients like Cipriano felt tended to and cared for in an increasingly corporatized medical system ingrained with structural racism.

I visited Perla one morning before she opened the door to patients like Cipriano and watched her set up the waiting room in her two-hundred-square-foot office, which she named La Plácita de la Salud.[1] "The fountain has two purposes," she told me, as she poured water into the topmost of the alternating stone pots that were hanging on her peach-colored wall. "One, because it is calming. I remember I liked it in the old doctor's office. The second is that it creates white noise. The walls here are paper-thin. You can hear everything." She was right. As soon as the water began trickling down, the acoustics in the room changed. "I wanted to create a homey atmosphere," said Perla. The compact front office doubled as a waiting room. She tidied up health pamphlets in Spanish and adjusted the colorful clay monarch butterflies hanging on the walls. A painting that read *"Aquí vive una médico"* [a doctor lives here] and her medical license also adorn the room.

Perla deliberately sought to practice in a way that differed from the norm. She sought to disrupt a medical training culture that privileged and reproduced white heteropatriarchal treatment plans with marginalized patients. She told me that she once shadowed a white male doctor who generalized about the "low pain tolerance" of immigrant Latino men. She remembered thinking, "That [attitude] doesn't help them want to see you. Who would want to continue seeing that doctor when you are at your most vulnerable? You want someone more sensitive. No berating or making you feel small." Indeed studies have shown that racial bias in pain management can result in inappropriate analgesic recommendations and affect patients' overall trust in the health-care system.[2] Confronting racial and ethnic bias was at the forefront of Perla's mind in the quality of care she provided.

Perla's start-up cost to set up a solo "micro practice" in a predominantly Spanish-speaking Latine community in southeastern Los Angeles was $10,000 in 2016. "I bought the most affordable furniture at IKEA [to fully furnish the entire space]," she mentioned. She also employed two medical assistants whom she interviewed, hired, and paid $18.00 an hour.[3] "I have everything I need here," she told me, beaming. "There is also a bathroom in the building so if a patient needs a urine test, I just send them there," instead of having to send them to another location.

Perla had recently acquired the office next door to make it a separate formal waiting room; the physical space was expanding to accommodate her growing patient base. The phones were usually ringing off the hook from patients scheduling appointments. Her husband, Salvador, a bilingual Mexican American man who served as her practice's clinical manager,[4] and Tessa, a young white medical assistant, shared the burden of answering them. I frequently heard Salvador follow "Doctor's office, this is Salvador speaking," with *"Buenos días, la razón por su visita?"* [Good morning. The reason for your visit?] It was also not unusual for Perla to schedule appointments when Salvador was out of the office. This would occur on days when their sitter was unavailable, and he had to handle the daytime needs of their toddler, as Tessa does not speak Spanish. Perla's schedule was regularly filled as she tended to the more than 850 patients, mostly of Mexican origin, who sought her care.[5] At the time of the interview, Perla was not accepting new patients, as she recognized she could not serve those she had if she did. Perla formed a private practice to buffer herself from gendered racism (as I showed in chapter 5) that she experienced in larger hospitals that systematically favored white physicians and patients.

Perla "centered the margins" in her practice by actively valuing the knowledge and perspectives of her patients, most of whom were working-class Latines. I argue that Latina/o doctors, who are mostly steered into or enter family and internal medicine, modify the quality of care they provide when serving the under-resourced sectors of the Latine community by blending biomedical science with their patients' sociocultural realities. Perla had set up her practice in as many ways as possible to enable this. The care Latina/o doctors want to provide Latine patients, however, is constrained by the health industry.

In this chapter, I take a *structural competency*[6] lens into medicine to present research grounded in the experiences and knowledges of patients of color with their physicians. Medical anthropologist and physician Seth Holmes examined the interactions of Oaxacan Triqui agricultural laborers with physicians in migrant health clinics located in Washington State and California.[7] Indigenous Triqui workers would frequently tell Holmes, *"los doctores no saben nada"* [doctors don't know anything] because physicians demonstrated little understanding of their Mexican indigenous cultures and of the quotidian structural violence they faced in their jobs. Some were self-medicating with alcohol to alleviate their pain to continue picking produce. Building on Holmes's work, I highlight patient counter-stories, foregrounding the experiences that are not always told or emphasized.[8] I also engage in a structural competency analysis. Different from culturally competent care, structural competency urges health-care professionals to think about how larger structural contexts shape patients' experiences at the intersection of race, class, gender, and ethnicity in a profit-driven health industry. This requires they recognize how social and economic determinants, biases, and inequities shape health and illness long before doctors and patients enter examination rooms.[9] Aleksandra Olszweski notes:

> When applied in medicine, counter-story can help to expose injustices and highlight the voices and experiences of patients and their families that might otherwise be missed or ignored. In doing so, this tool can help clinicians both recognize racism and other systems of oppression in their work and explor[e] [a] patient's or family's unique experience or perspective in order to provide individualized, co-feeling care.[10]

I draw from select ethnographic vignettes with sixteen doctor-patient visits to highlight how patients describe their ailments, and the individual interviews I conducted illuminate how Latina/o doctors respond, interact, and care for them.[11] Counter-stories, in conjunction with a structural competency perspective that Latina/o physicians engage in, are salient to providing care in small private practices, community clinics, and large hospitals. Equity work happened both within and across organizations for bilingual Latina/o physicians.

## CENTERING THE MARGINS WITH PATIENT COUNTER-STORIES

When I came to observe Perla's interactions with her patients, Tessa was at the receptionist's table working on the computer. At 12:31 p.m. the doorbell rang, signaling that a patient was waiting to be buzzed in. This was the first time I saw Cipriano. An older man, he was wearing blue Wrangler jeans and a white shirt with a puffer vest. As he entered the waiting room, Tessa said, "I'm gonna take your blood pressure." She had his record up on an iPad and recorded the results of the blood-pressure cuff, pulse oximeter, forehead thermometer, and digital scale.[12] Tessa conducts intake and inputs patients' vitals in the system in a corner of the waiting room; there is a small nook where she measures height and weight. "Is high?" Cipriano asked in English about his blood pressure. "I'm gonna have the doctor explain that," she whispered. Cipriano took a seat in the waiting room, where I was also waiting, after the measurements were complete.

Perla came out of her office within a minute and greeted Cipriano. She informed him that I was a *profesora de UCI* and was there to observe Latina/o doctors and their interactions with patients. She asked him if I might observe the visit and informed him that I was not going to record any identifying information. He agreed with a jovial smile. Cipriano told me that he initially thought I was another patient. Perla escorted him in, and he sat on a white plastic chair beside the examination table.

Cipriano was sixty-nine years old and had a terrible cough. Through coughs that he was trying to restrain, he said, *"Tengo tres días con tos que no me puedo dormir. Siento irritado. He tomado jarabe y nada. Me duele mi pecho."* [I have had a cough for three days that won't let me sleep. My throat feels irritated. I drank cough syrups and nothing. My chest hurts.][13]

Perla assured him, *"Está bien si tose."* [It is fine if you cough.] Suppressing his cough and trying to swallow the phlegm was causing him discomfort. Noticing that the patient was in pain when he put his arms on his chest and hunched over to cough into his curled-up hand, Perla had him remove his vest in the chair instead of having him step up onto the examination table so she could listen to his lungs. It was a small measure to put his comfort over her convenience that I noticed immediately. Perla placed the stethoscope on his back, asking him to take deep breaths. She then examined his throat, putting on blue latex gloves before inserting a tongue depressor into his mouth.

As she typed notes into the computer, Cipriano raised his arm above his head, bent it up and down, and rotated it round and round to show his regained mobility. *"Mire doctora, se me quito el dolor del brazo. Ire!"*[14] [Look doctor, my arm pain went away. Look!] Perla filled me in: he had come in a couple of months before with a sharp pain in his shoulder, which she noted was a rotator cuff injury.

Presumably for my benefit, Cipriano showered praise on Perla's practice. He talked about how difficult it was to get an appointment in other locations and that it was simpler for him to see Perla because he did not have to deal with an automated system or press numbers on the phone. He was able to reach an actual person in her micro-clinic and said he felt *"a gusto,"* or comfortable receiving care there. Several studies have noted that Spanish-speaking immigrants are often told by staff that they should take whatever appointment is offered to them regardless of their schedules because they are poor, and that this affects their continuity of care. At times they wait over two hours to be seen by a provider, particularly when they are lower income.[15]

Perla told the patient that she was going to give him something stronger for his infection than what he was taking. *"Le voy a dar pastillas para el dolor de pecho para la infección. Necesita algo mas agresivo. Le voy a recomendar una pica."* [I am going to give you pills for the pain in your chest for the infection. You need something more aggressive. I'm going to recommend an injection.] He rolled up his right sleeve to ready his arm for the shot as she prepared the syringe with the solution.

Cipriano revealed that he took the bus to his appointment. Most of Perla's patients, I learned, walked or took public transportation, though one patient, the mother of an infant, drove nearly two hours to get a referral to an ophthalmologist from Perla. The woman had to pay for a sitter for her infant and the doctors to whom Perla could confidently refer her were also near Perla's practice, a fact Perla lamented to me. I assumed that the Spanish-language name of Perla's practice might have made the drive seem worth it to the patient, but Perla suspected the insurance provider, Aetna, had given her few options.

Whether it was work schedules, relying on a relative for a ride, or missing an appointment due to bus driver strikes, simply getting to the appointment was a concern for patients. I saw Salvador's sensitivity to this issue when he found an hour-long block for a married couple so that they could travel together instead of taking separate trips to see Perla.

Perla escorted Cipriano back into the waiting room so he could check out with Tessa, but she told me I could remain in the examination room to debrief. When she returned, Perla told me that sometimes patients go across the US-Mexico border to places like Tijuana because they prefer receiving injections as a form of treatment. "Everything is an injection. It is a treatment they recognize from childhood. They think they get an antibiotic, but it is an anti-inflammatory. They leave already feeling better." Sociologist Danielle Raudenbush indicates that some Mexican immigrants engage in cross-border health-seeking behaviors to achieve what they believe to be optimal health-care results.[16] This happens when US doctors will not prescribe certain pharmaceuticals or when patients are dissatisfied with their care. Before finding Perla's practice, Cipriano engaged in this type of medical tourism.

Culturally competent care, in which providers and the organizations for which they work meet the social and cross-cultural linguistic needs of diverse patients, is difficult to find, and Cipriano was visibly glad he had found it. The US federal government has required that medical practitioners provide culturally competent care since 2001. The Department of Health and Human Services provides a list of fourteen individual national standards that comprise Cultural and Linguistically Appropriate Services (CLAS) in health care. One standard states, "Healthcare organizations must assure the competence of language assistance provided to limited English proficient patients/consumers by interpreters and bilingual staff. Family and friends should not be used to provide interpretation services (except on request by the patient)."[17] While a medical interpreter should always be present, many organizations are not meeting this standard, and children are often tasked with performing this labor for immigrant parents.[18] These standards are intended to make services more responsive to the individual needs of patients from diverse backgrounds, to ensure continuity of care, and to avoid misdiagnoses or omission of vital information. More often than not, however, the children of immigrants drive their parents to appointments to ensure that their loved one's concerns are not minimized and to advocate for them. Rosa, who opened this book, regularly did this for her father.

Minda was also clearly grateful to receive culturally competent care. I returned to the waiting room until she gave permission for me to be present for her consultation. As she was filling out her forms, she asked me in Spanish if I knew the date, and I replied in Spanish. *"Día 15, mes 7,"* she said as she jotted it down.[19] She then asked me if I was a patient, and I told her that I was there to observe patients and their interactions with Perla. I was the only other person in the waiting room. Without hesitation, continuing to talk to me as Tessa took her vitals, Minda shared, *"Yo me siento bien. Me puedo comunicar en español. Prefiero español. No quiero traer a mis hijos para que me traduzcan. El directorio de MediCal dice los [doctores] de español. Es muy bonito tener un doctor que habla español."* [I feel good (here). I can communicate in Spanish. I prefer Spanish. I don't want to bring my children to interpret. The MediCal directory tells you which doctors speak Spanish. It is beautiful to have a Spanish-speaking physician.]

Perla had told me that Minda might be a little upset with her because she had called over the weekend seeking antibiotics and had been forced to go to the emergency room. The office was closed over the weekend, but I did not see any sign of being upset in her demeanor. Like Cipriano, she cheerfully permitted me to join her in Perla's office. When the doctor asked, *"¿Cómo se siente? Malita?"* [How do you feel? Unwell?], Minda described how she had gone to the ER because she was having difficulty breathing and was vomiting. She was worried because her throat hurt, and she feared it would close. She voluntarily shared that at the ER, she was treated by a white woman doctor who had a Latino nurse interpret for her. *"El me entendió y me ayudaron. Me sacaron el pipí y me dieron inyección en cada pompa."* [He understood me, and they helped me. They got a urine sample and gave me an injection in each glute.] The woman had received amoxicillin and an allergy medication. While these measures had helped, concerns remained. She said, *"Lo que me da miedo es que yo tenga rota la nariz y nomas [sic] respiro con un lado."* [What scares me is that my nose may be torn; I can only breathe through one side.] She pushed her functioning nostril with her index finger and attempted to breathe with the other one to show the doctor that it was blocked. She continued, *"Se me entumen las manos y unos me dicen que tengo mala circulación."* [My hands get numb, and some people tell me I have bad circulation.]

Perla observed, *"Eso no es por la nariz."* [That's not because of your nose.] Rather than diminishing the patient's culturally inflected understanding of her syndromes, Perla informed her that the nose obstruction was separate from the wear and tear on her hands and legs due to her job and recommended she see a specialist.

Minda continued, *"Tengo miedo. La doctora gringa dijo que me tenía que hacer cirugía. No he podido dormir."* [I am afraid. The white doctor said they had to do surgery. I haven't been able to sleep.] She had an inhaler, but it caused her to cough.

*"¿No le dieron jarabes? ¿Le puedo dar un jarabe?"* [Have they prescribed cough syrups? I can give you a syrup], said Perla.

The woman had tried everything, but nothing worked. She felt that her job had exacerbated her condition. *"Trabajo en un lugar muy frío y hay mucho polvo porque trabajo en una lavandería."* [I work in a very cold place and there is a lot of dust because I work in a laundromat.] Minda revealed she had previously worked as a housekeeper but that the chemicals and backache made it impossible to continue. Perla said she would give the patient a referral for an ear, nose, and throat doctor.

A report based on surveying one hundred New York City laundromats suggests that Minda's belief that her work was making her sick is likely accurate. The report found that few workers were aware they needed to use protective equipment such as gloves or facial masks to protect themselves from the effects of breathing in industrial soaps or when cleaning dust in large dryers that may not be equipped with high-efficiency particulate air filters.[20] Those workers, mostly immigrant women of color like Minda, reported muscle pain, allergies, and skin conditions. Some had respiratory problems similar to Minda's.

Perla examined Minda's throat. *"A ver, digame ahhh"* [Let me see], she said, as she put the tongue depressor in the patient's mouth. Perla said that it did look very irritated.

Minda said, *"Siento como unas bolotas"* [I feel these large ball-shaped obstructions], and told her about her experience in the emergency room over the weekend. *"Fue muy buena la doctora."* [She was a good doctor.]

Perla asked the patient to lie down. *"¿La alhmuada esta buena?"* [Is the pillow fine?]

*"Para mí, muy buena"* [Really good for me], Minda said as she rested her head on the pillow.

Perla noted that Minda's ankles were very swollen from standing at work all day. Then she instructed, *"Esta libre, la autorización le va a llegar por el correo."* [You are free. You will receive the authorization (to see an otolaryngologist) in the mail.] Perla gave her a referral to an otolaryngologist to see if they could better examine her airways and diagnose her respiratory condition.

When the patient left, Perla explained to me that many of the Latina/o immigrant patients she cared for had "over-use" musculoskeletal injuries, caused by repetitive movements in their manual jobs. A report by the Pew Research Center notes that Latina/o adults explain that working in jobs with health risks is the top factor for their poorer health outcomes than other US adults.[21] Perla is quite different from the clinicians in Seth Holmes's study, who worked in severely under-resourced migrant clinics and very rarely asked questions about the living or working conditions of their migrant patients.[22] She is far more like those in a study by Ivy Torres and colleagues, who would provide paperwork so that patients could compel their employers to give them work breaks to take needed insulin.[23] Perla listened to her patients, and she also knew the descriptors patients used to describe their ailments. Some patients described their ailments using cultural-typical phrases such as *mala circulación* [bad blood circulation] or *entumido* [numbness]. Perla told me that bad blood circulation is "not really a thing," but that she understands what patients are describing: "When patients stand for hours and hours that happens. It could be a pinched nerve, or something else." Perla explained that her patients have difficulty getting sick leave and that this worsens their injuries. Perla's understanding of the sociocultural context of her patients' work, Spanish-language fluency, and cultural and structural competency are now critical skills for accurately diagnosing people and providing care.

## BLAMING THE PATIENT'S CULTURE

The majority of the physicians I interviewed exhibited different degrees of cultural competency, and many explained that some of their coworkers and medical resident trainees blamed Latine immigrant patients for their ailments or brushed away their concerns. Even well-intentioned culturally competent curricula at times mobilize stereotypes of people of color in efforts to diagnose behavioral choices as likely causes of health disparities. This pathologizes patient populations and omits a deeper analysis of systemic forces that create environments within which people exert autonomy and make their choices under greatly constrained conditions.[24] Indeed, most mainstream cultural competency training focuses on a list of stereotypical traits of ethnic groups,[25] essentializing and homogenizing Latine cultures. Mainstream cultural competency training often assumes the culture of the patient is the problem that needs to be understood and a barrier that can and should be overcome. The Triqui migrant patients in Seth Holmes's study referenced both structural obstacles to care and the perceptions and presumptions of their health-care providers as equally contributing to their failure to receive health care. The mostly white clinicians Holmes interviewed and observed saw undocumented Triqui migrants as more respectful than white patients, tough, and deserving of quality health care. At the same time, they saw them as frustrating due to their "traditional" health beliefs and vague medical histories.[26]

Evidence suggests Latine cultural beliefs are not well understood among service providers in the American health-care delivery system[27] in ways similar to the Hmong immigrant family in Anne Fadiman's book *The Spirit Catches You and You Fall Down: A Hmong Child, Her American Doctors, and the Collision of Two Cultures.*[28] While the biomedical condition the young child in title suffers from is epileptic seizures, the book shows how an understanding of cultural differences can effectively promote positive health outcomes. When patients have someone who understands their ailments, they gain comfort and connection and develop the *confianza* to explain more about their conditions and needs. Holmes argues that the structure and culture of biomedicine form the primary barriers to effective care as they prevent medical professionals from seeing the social determinants of the suffering of their unauthorized patients.[29] Medical scholars suggest that clinicians must unlearn how they are taught about race in medical training to see race as a social construct.[30] Otherwise, they may feel little sympathy for patients. They may think that, as the doctors in *Boys in White* did in the 1950s, that "patients who do not follow medical advice more or less deserve what they get" or that they "become diseased as a consequence of their own action or neglect."[31] *Boys in White* described such thinking among white men medical students. Social class culture seemed to furnish the basis for complaints that "charity patients" did not act properly as "poor" or submissive. These ideas still linger in medicine's culture today, as the Latina/o physicians told me during the individual interviews.

In my previous work on Latina elementary school teachers, I coined the term "Chicana/Latina cultural pedagogies" to describe how Spanish-speaking Latina teachers were able to subtly modify their interactional modes in response to language cues exhibited by Latine immigrant parents. They did this to generate comfort and ease in the classroom or in parent-teacher meetings without relying on children to serve as interpreters or cultural brokers. They described an understanding of conversational etiquette that made it possible for them to establish rapport with Spanish-speaking parents.[32]

Some bilingual and bicultural Latina/o physicians exhibited similar modifications. Medical Spanish requires knowing the technical terminology that I was fortunate enough to study at El Instituto Cultural Oaxaca,[33] as well as the more common lay terms that ordinary people use. Soraida, the Puerto Rican heritage physician introduced in the previous chapter, explained that patients used words such as *picazón* [stabbing pain], *dolor en el pecho* [pain in the chest], *susto* [fright], *coyunturas* [joints], *culebrilla* [shingles], *bilis* [digestive issues], or *agruras* [heartburn] to describe their ailments. Soraida did her due diligence as a physician and looked up *agruras* because she had never heard it before.[34] The Spanish language is not uniform, and Latina/o physicians often made additional attempts to comprehend diverse sociocultural ailments. Other patients would use cultural expressions such as ¡*"me dolió hasta el corazón o el alma!"* [it hurt me to the core] to signal the severity of their pain, or *mal de ojo* [the evil eye] to signify an unexplained ailment. Ignacio, a Mexican origin doctor in family medicine, told me about these phrases; he understood that when patients used them they did not mean that they were having heart or eye problems. When cultural metaphors are not compatible with biomedical concepts or not congruent with clinical expectations, a lack of communication between physician and patient is common.[35]

Perla's bridging of cultural metaphors and biomedical concepts was particularly evident during Eugenia's visit. Eugenia spoke about a swishing sound in her ear. *"Cuando estornudo siento agua. Me pongo agua tibia, lo que me hacía mi abuelita. Antes tenia sangre. Me lave el oido. No es dolor nomas [sic] una molestia."* [When I sneeze, I feel water. I put warm water in my ear, what my grandmother would do to me. Before I had blood. I cleaned my ear. It is not pain, just a nuisance.]

Perla asked Eugenia if she had ever used drops in her ear or if she had injured it. *"¿Puede ser que tiene cicatriz en el timpani?"* [It could be that you have a scar in your tensor tympani muscle].

The woman listed several treatments she had tried, including a folk remedy like lighting a candlestick or a newspaper on fire and putting one end in her auditory canal. Ear candling or coning is believed to relieve earaches but is also associated with considerable risks such as burns.[36] Alongside her ear problem she also said that her neck was tense.

Perla touched her neck and massaged each side. *"Usted lo que tiene es artritis en el mandibular. Entonces no es el oido, es el artritis."* [What you have is arthritis in your mandible. So, it is not your ear, it is arthritis.] This made sense to the patient because she often felt discomfort or cracking when she chewed.

Of the care she received from Perla, this patient revealed, *"Es más que el lenguaje. Es el poder hablar con ella."* [It's more than just speaking Spanish. It is the ability to be able to talk to her.][37] Such remarks reflect the fact that Perla works to avoid victim blaming and cultural racism, much like Thalia. Thalia, the daughter of Mexican immigrants, noted that some of her non-Latina/o physician coworkers labeled patients as noncompliant when they could not get patients to follow their directives. Thalia, in internal medicine, told me that her colleagues do not recognize that patients who do not follow treatment may be nonadherent instead of noncompliant. They may be confused or overwhelmed and therefore unable to comply with a treatment plan. Thalia noted that some physicians would label Latine Spanish-speaking immigrant patients as noncompliant because they were having a "hard time analyzing" the patient. Thalia recalled one notable case with an elderly patient named Mrs. Vega:

I know Mrs. Vega very well. . . . I tell them [the doctors], 'Did you get a translator?' They answer, 'No.' I ask them, 'Are you being coherent? Is she being cognitively impaired?' They say, 'No.' Then, I tell them, 'Mrs. Vega is [sharp]. She knows exactly what medicine she's on, how much she's on when it got started, what doctor gave it to her, and for what reason. If you're telling me that she is not compliant, you better get a translator because that word does not exist for her. This eighty-one-year-old woman is sharp, and if you can't get a history from her, you need to try again.' Culturally speaking, the fact that they don't speak English, assumptions get made about their level of intelligence, awareness about their medical conditions and the medications they're on, and their understanding of the process.

Thalia noted that the lack of language-competent care caused some physicians and staff to blame patients for their conditions and question their cognitive abilities. This was also evident when a Latina immigrant woman in her fifties wearing a red suit, red shoes, and red lipstick arrived at Perla's office. *"Buenos dias,* Good morning," the woman said, laughing in my direction. *"Para que no digan que no soy bilingüe"* [So they don't say I'm not bilingual], she said to me. I gathered that the patient knew her language abilities (as well as her attire) might affect how people treated her, and she greeted everyone in both languages as a preventive measure.

Rocío, a rheumatologist who worked in a large hospital in Los Angeles, noted similar patterns in her specialty. She conveyed,

> There tends to be less patience and compassion from white doctors and other minority groups [Asian] with this patient population. There is that kind of stereotypical joke of the Latina woman or old grandma that comes in with pain, '*ay ay ay ay!*' [ouch or ow]. We see that a lot here [and] attention sometimes isn't paid. I'm not going to say that I'm completely innocent of that but because of where I come from [Amarillo, Texas], I understand it a little better. As a consequence, I have more patience and compassion.

Amarillo is the most populous city in the Texas Panhandle with a large concentration of Latine and white residents. Rocío described that some non-Latino physicians in the large hospital she worked at would poke fun at the way that Latines expressed their pain, minimizing it. She talked about the importance of cultural humility. Cultural humility goes beyond cultural competence in that it recognizes institutional barriers and acknowledges power imbalances between clinicians and patients.[38] Cultural competence may encourage physicians to understand culture as an explanatory variable, encouraging them to stereotype and essentialize their minority patients. Attempting to level power imbalances means that physicians need to be reflexive about their power, privilege, and prejudices to challenge any implicit biases they may have about people or have learned in traditional medical school curricula.

Rosa described witnessing cultural racism toward Latine patients, especially when residents in training were in a rush. She observed:

> I see it with the residents, not necessarily white. There's been African American, Asian, even Latines. It's hard work [in residency]. They're really busy and sometimes they don't understand where the patient's coming from. It's really easy to judge and say, 'I don't understand, this patient's crazy. Why won't they just take their medications?' You have to step back

and say, 'You said the patient's crazy. Is the patient really crazy? Is there some mental health issue going on?' They respond, 'No, they are just not compliant with their medication.' I say, 'Well don't label them as crazy. They're not. Are they noncompliant with their medication? Let's explore that. Why are they noncompliant? Are they not getting it? Did they not bring their bottles? Do they know they need to bring their medication? Is it too many medications? Maybe we need to cut down treatment and explain it. Have you given them a written list? Have you asked them to bring the written list?' Those are the things you must do. But the residents—because I worked with them so closely, they get so frustrated.

Similarly, Olivia explained what she witnessed during clinical rounds:

I can be in clinical rounds, and they are talking about a family not being compliant. They were trying to get medications in the home. I said, 'Are you making sure that the nurse that is going to the home to help this family who has never had cancer or any other medical illness? You're expecting this family to give IV medicines through a line, shots in the leg, and all of this? Did you even think about getting or asking a nurse who was Spanish-speaking if they were a monolingual Spanish family?' I say, 'Why are you not thinking about this? You are worried about compliance but what if someone talked to you in Russian? Would you be able to do it? No!'

Unfortunately, Rocío, Rosa, and Olivia—who all worked in various hospitals in Los Angeles—get at the enforcement of the magic fifteen-minute appointments during medical training. This is not a structure that is conducive to listening, paying attention to a patient, and trying to see it their way. All attempted to train the residents who worked with them to examine the root of what was causing misunderstandings to occur. At times patients described that they did not take their medications properly for weeks. They did not understand the directions that the pharmacy provided because they were written in English.

Rosa recalled a teachable moment she had experienced:

I had another resident. She wasn't Latina. She was talking about obesity in Latine patients. She's like, 'Oh, this patient is so fat!' I told her 'That's not very sensitive. You need to be careful how to talk about patients. . . . It's disrespectful.' The resident was very embarrassed. Apologetically she responded, 'You're completely right.' Teaching that sensitivity is not easy. [A lot] of times it's because [patients are] not eating well.

Olivia and Rosa must address these issues instead of letting them slide and giving the inadvertent impression that these comments are acceptable. Rosa also alluded to the lack of availability of nutritious food in certain communities that have been priced out of attaining it due to food insecurity, food deserts, or food swamps. Cultural and medical anthropologist Alysha Gálvez argues that modernization and globalization have created systems that make people more susceptible to developing chronic diseases like diabetes.[39] Many Latina/o physicians are now treating patients affected by this form of structural change in their diets. Ethan, a multiracial Puerto Rican and white family medicine doctor, explained that the "number one diagnosis" in his office was "chronic diabetes and obesity" and also noted that physicians would not recommend certain foods to Latine patients. He explained,

Diet and attitudes toward exercise are unique in Latino culture[s]. It doesn't mean that every Latino has diabetes and is obese, but we know, statistically, that they have a higher rate, and diet contributes to that. It's a culturally bound value that's pretty hard to get away from completely. Kale and quinoa—I haven't heard those things recommended to my patients. . . . You have to start where patients are, and maybe just reduce *pan dulce* in the morning from three pieces to one.

While Ethan's words may appear to veer dangerously close to culturally deficient assumptions by supposing his patients are merely overeating sweets, he works to help patients modify their diets rather than extirpating it all. He also recognizes that certain foods may not be available to Latine patients. I found in my study of Latina teachers that women were more adept at addressing cultural nuances with Latine families because they were more likely to perform this interpretation work early on. In medicine, however, bilingual men engaged in these practices too.

Latina/o doctors regularly mentioned the difficulties of addressing diet with patients. A consultation I saw with a middle-aged Latino man in which he and his doctor discussed blood test results showing he was borderline diabetic suggests how poorly this can go when doctors do not understand the context. The patient explained that he thought working in construction was exercise. Not seeming to hear, the physician drew the man a picture of a plate with portions devoted to different types of foods and told him that he needed to exercise to the point of panting. The doctor seemed unaware of the cultural aspects of food and that the man's working hours and conditions did not allow him time for dedicated strenuous exercise, except on occasional weekends when he could play soccer. Mauricio, who worked in critical care for a large HMO near California's Silicon Valley, remembered how his Mexican immigrant father thought some of the foods he was eating were healthy and didn't know they could affect him. "There's a culture gap. My dad didn't understand the basics of diabetes. There was something that was missing that we couldn't know. Like, 'Oh, my God bread is bad for you, tortillas are bad for you.' That kind of made me learn about this disease and educate him and start teaching him." Like many young aspiring Latina/o physicians who frequently had these encounters with family members,[40] Mauricio realized that so many others would also benefit from having this medical knowledge.

Type 2 diabetes—a chronic condition that affects how the body processes glucose—has resulted in a public health emergency in both Latin America and the United States. The traditional "milpa-based diet"—a corn-centered diet—has been affected by globalization and changed peoples' abilities to access certain foods at affordable costs.[41] Karen, who worked for a large medical center in LA County, described how cultural competence in helping patients manage diabetes affects her interactions with them:

> When I am explaining to them about their diet I tell them, 'I know you are used to eating *arroz* [rice] and *frijoles* [beans] and *carne* [meat] and tortillas.' This is what your plate looks like, and this is what it should look like. I let them fill in what it should look like. Half of it has to be veggies. 'Tell me how you're going to do that.' You approach it that way. You're coming from a point of, 'I just want to help you. I am not here to punish, reprimand, or tell you how bad you are.'

Instead of asking patients to merely buy expensive foods like "organic quinoa" Karen would provide nutrition educational activities during office visits. Studies have found an association between provider diabetes management behaviors and patient race. While Black patients were least likely to be counseled on dietary changes, physical changes, or adjustments made by primary care providers to their medication,[42] here we see how some Latina/o doctors implemented cultural competence in diabetes management.

## ENGAGING IN STRUCTURALLY COMPETENT CARE

Social determinants of health such as economic, social, and legal conditions, have influenced multiple disease outcomes among immigrant families that also go beyond diabetes, and may result from allostatic load. Stressors like family separation, acculturation, stigmatization, and dangerous border crossings accumulate and afflict immigrants in distinct ways. Some endure Immigrant Syndrome with Chronic and Multiple Stress (also known as *síndrome Ulises* [Ulysses Syndrome]),[43] which physicians either address or ignore.

Lisa, who worked at a teaching hospital in an urban location, also blended biomedical science with her patients' sociocultural realities and socioeconomic constraints. She had to contend with structural obstacles beyond her control that materialized for her in ways much different than for Perla at her micro-clinic. I came to observe Lisa on her last day treating patients at a small Catholic-funded clinic in a low-income area twenty miles south of Los Angeles.[44] Most of the patients at this facility were undocumented, did not qualify for coverage under the Affordable Care Act, and primarily spoke Spanish. Lisa had been there for five years, having replaced another Latina doctor who had left for a position at a managed care organization. Now Lisa had taken a new job with a bigger research hospital in Los Angeles.

Lisa was overseeing three different interns and sending them into different patient rooms after each intern presented her with the case and their proposed course of action. One of the interns was Pushpa, a South Asian woman who was going to medical school in Arizona but doing her rotations in California. "I just met Pushpa today," Lisa told me. With the permission of the patient, I watched a visit with Lisa, Pushpa, and a patient who does not speak English.

Lisa mentioned that she doesn't like to translate, but that she would do so for Pushpa to help her learn, and she began the visit by saying, *"Tengo a dos visitantes conmigo. Esta bien si estan en el cuarto? Todas somos mujeres."* [I have two visitors with me. It is okay if they are in the room? We are all women.]

"*Si, esta bien*" [Yes, that's all right], the woman replied.

"*¿Usted habla español?*"—the patient asked me if I spoke Spanish.

"*Sí*," I responded.

"*A ella no le pregunto por que se que no sabe*" [I won't ask her because I know she doesn't know], the woman said, pointing toward Pushpa with her chin.

Pushpa interjected in English, "I can understand it but can't speak it."

I interpreted, *"Dice que si lo entiende."* [She says she can understand it.]

The woman answered, *"He visto muchos de esos doctores y saben hablar el español bien."* [I've seen many of those [South Asian] doctors and they know how to speak Spanish well.] Delfina was a middle-aged Latina. She had visited the clinic a couple of days before for a pregnancy test. The test came back negative, but she remained suspicious she was pregnant because her breast had a clear discharge. Pushpa asked her a series of questions regarding her sexual history and Lisa interpreted everything back and forth. I wondered if I should continue the task I had started but that didn't capture the daily lived realities for Latina/o doctors who find themselves in this position with coworkers and trainees.

Lisa nonetheless asked me how to say "nipple." When I could not recall the word for the anatomical part in Spanish fast enough, Lisa said, "*¿Cómo se dice?*" [How do you say?] to the patient and pointed to her nipple.

The patient understood. "*Nosotros le decimos pezón en mi país. Tambien puede ser tetilla o engrasador.*" [We say *pezón* in my country. It can also be *tetilla* or *engrasador*.]

"*Ah, sí! ¿De dónde es usted?*" [Oh, yes. Where are you from?], Lisa responded.

"*Yo soy del Salvador.*" [I'm from El Salvador.]

"*Yo también soy Salvadoreña. Me acuerdo que de ese modo se dice.*" [I am also Salvadoran. I remember that's how you say it.]

Lisa was called out of the room by one of the nurses, and Pushpa asked me if I would interpret. I said I would do my best. I successfully translated an interaction in which Pushpa learned that the patient's breast was tender and that the discharge was clear. Then Lisa returned, and they asked the woman to undress from the waist up and put on a gown. The patient obliged. "*Todas somos mujeres, ¿verdad?*" [We are all women, right?] she said, because there would be three people in the room, rather than just her and one provider.[45]

When we re-entered the room so that the providers could give the woman a breast exam, Lisa touched the woman's right breast and told Pushpa, "You can do that breast." I listened as Lisa told Pushpa what to feel for and as she imparted the information to Delfina.

After the exam, Delfina asked if she could get birth control at this facility if she was not pregnant. Lisa interpreted and turned to Pushpa, "Do you know the answer to that?"

"No," she replied.

"At this facility, you cannot because it is Catholic," Lisa answered. She turned to the patient and communicated, *"En esta clínica no le puedo dar eso. Si estuviera en otra clínica si se lo daría porque yo pienso que es importante. Pero la puedo mandar a otro lugar para que las consiga."* [I cannot give you (birth control) in this facility. If I were in another clinic, I would give it to you because I think it is important. But I can send you to another place where you can obtain it.]

Lisa had told me that she had found a new job in part because she was unhappy with such limitations. It also paid more.

The free clinic also did not provide school immunizations because those had to be done at the county, as she told an undocumented Mexican immigrant mother who was seeking them for her four-year-old son to enroll him in school. Looking at the floor, the mother said, *"Es que cuando cruzamos no traje los documentos de las vacunas. A él lo trajimos a los dos años. Le pusiero dos vacunas [en México]. Lo traje por que dijeron que necesita vacunas par ir a la escuela."* [When we crossed (the border) I did not bring the immunization document. We brought him at two years old. He received his vaccinations in Mexico. I brought him because they said he needed inoculations to go to school.][46]

*"No necesitan documentos,"* Lisa reassured the woman as she directed her elsewhere for the vital preventive care for her son.

Lisa's frustrations at the clinic manifested with most of the patients that she saw, and most, if not all, were due to structural limitations imposed by the health industry. Finding locations that had the necessary equipment or machines was a struggle for Latina/o doctors who were trying to advocate for their patients. This was the case for another patient that I observed who needed x-rays on her knee; it was only *"por chiripazo, por coincidencia"* [sheer luck] that she was able to get an appointment near her hometown of Montebello. This patient had been involved in a car accident and was sent to a facility in East LA. She called for over a month to get an appointment with no luck and later learned that the MRI machine had broken down. In our one-on-one interview, Benito pointed to a brown paper bag on his work shelf to indicate where he recycled his N95 mask in a small attempt to save resources for the disenfranchised patients in two Latine ethnic enclaves he treated who had limited access to them during COVID-19 and who had to keep working as essential laborers or lived-in high-density neighborhoods.[47] Benito got visibly teary-eyed when recounting the effects that the novel coronavirus had on his own extended family and the disparities in resource and information dissemination, a topic I address in the afterword. It was up to Latina/o doctors to find resources for patients when resources were paltry, placing a significant strain on their shoulders.

Lisa's interactions with her next patient, Fidel, exemplify the emotional weight Latinas/os manage while caring for co-ethnic patients. Fidel was an older immigrant man who arrived at the visit with his wife. Lisa informed him that Fernie, a student who was pursuing an MA in biology at CSU-Fullerton, and I would both be in the room. The patient indicated this was acceptable, but he asked why we wanted to observe. Fernie said that he wanted to shadow Lisa because he wanted to be a nurse. I said that I was writing a book about Latina/o physicians. Fidel followed up, *"¿Es para ayudarnos? ¿Para quedar bien?"* [Is it to help us? (meaning Latinos). To make a good impression (on me)?] We all laughed.

*"¿Cómo se siente?"* [How do you feel?], Lisa asked.

Shakily, Fidel responded, *"Un poquito mejor."* [A little better.]

Lisa said that he looked better. The last time he was in the clinic he had been hunched over, and his gait was abnormal, as if he were taking baby steps. At the time he thought he had a kidney problem. Lisa turned to a screen that was mounted onto the wall and displayed the human body's internal organs. She zoomed in on the image and showed the patient and his wife what was going on with his intestines. His wife listened intently. She was worried.

"*Usted tiene una hernia en los intestinos*" [You have a hernia in your intestines], Lisa said, pointing to it.

"Oh," the man and his wife said in unison.

Lisa explained, "*Si tuviera aseguranza lo mandaría con un cirujano de hernia. Pero eso no es opción. No tiene aseguranza sino lo mandaría con un especialista.*" [If you had insurance, I would send you to a hernia surgeon. But that is not an option. You don't have insurance, if not I would send you to a specialist.][48]

Fidel shook his head no and inquired, "*¿Cuánto cuesta? ¿No se puede pagar en efectivo?*" [How much does it cost? Can we pay with cash?] in hopes that the family could raise the money. Lisa informed him it would cost $300-$400 to look at one part of the body. "*Usted necesita un MRI*" [You need an MRI], Lisa told him, because she worried about possible strangulation, a more serious problem.

"*Y somos pobrecitos nosotros*" [And we are poor], Fidel laughed nervously.

Fidel, his wife, and Lisa herself were aware of the financial limitations he faced. Lisa wanted to provide more aid than she possibly could. She had become a family medicine doctor in the first place because she wanted to work for a marginalized Latine community. With hesitancy, she proposed, "*Le puedo recomendar ejercisio para más fuerza o más medicina. Podemos tratar con un cirujano. Hay un cirujano en Los Angeles pero no se si usted pueda ir para alla*" [I can recommend some exercises to strengthen your muscles or more medication. We can try with a surgeon. There is a surgeon in Los Angeles, but I don't know if you can go over there.] She was hoping she could connect Fidel with one of her new networks at the hospital where she would be working and with someone who could see Fidel even though he didn't have insurance. Unsure if he could find transportation to Los Angeles, she asked him, "*¿Qué hacemos?*" [What do we do?]

*"Esperarme"* [Wait], the patient responded despondently. His shoulders sank. It seemed that waiting to see if the doctor's office in Los Angeles would contact him so that he could see a specialist was his only option.

Fidel had other matters to discuss while he waited for a chance to address his hernia. *"Otra cosa, doctora."* [Another thing, doctor]. He pulled a blood-pressure cuff out of his bag, saying that he had obtained extremely high readings and thought he was probably using it incorrectly. Lisa instructed him in measuring his blood pressure, giving the patient far more time than we would have expected. Lisa thought this was important to do because she wanted to ensure all his many health-related concerns (high blood pressure, diabetes, and intestinal hernia) were answered before she left the clinic. Then Fidel pulled out some supplements that he had purchased at a *botánica*, saying that he had heard from people in his community that they would help him with his conditions. Lisa told him that she did not have training in vitamin supplements and that perhaps he should save his money, but she also noted that if a pill didn't make his hernia swell and he felt all right, it might make sense to take it for the placebo effect.

Fidel also indicated that he was confused about his medication because it changed constantly. Some of his medicines were not renewed at the pharmacy and he did not understand why.

Lisa looked at his chart. *"Vienen tantos doctores y todos miran algo diferente. Este le bajó la medicina. No fui yo. Aquí dice que según le quitaron. Esta tomando la medicina de la próstata?"* [So many doctors come, and they all see something different. This one lowered your dosage. It wasn't me. Here it says that they removed [the medication]. Are you taking the medicine for your prostate?] The patient indicated he was. In contrast to the "extremely patchy" medical records that clinicians in Holmes's study lamented concerning their seasonal migrant worker patients,[49] Fidel's file was full, but it had contradictory information filled out by the various clinicians who cycled through the facility. Working in this small organization accelerated the burnout Lisa was feeling.

Lisa instructed Fidel, *"La próxima vez que venga traiga todas sus medicinas. Es important que se tome esta. Es para que no le de ataque de corazón o un derrame cerebral. Nomas [sic] se tiene que tomar una para la presión."* [The next time you come bring all of your medications. You must take this one. It's so that you don't get a heart attack or a stroke. You only need to take one for the pressure.] Lisa was trying to compensate for the practice's weakness—caused by frequent turnover—by informing the patient that he might have been taking too many medicines to control his blood pressure.

The patient said that he tried a new pharmacy because he was hoping he would be able to get all of his medications that way. *"En dos meses no me dieron insulina"* [In two months they didn't give me insulin], he shared. He had been without it for those two months.

Lisa looked frustrated. It is dangerous for Fidel to stop taking his insulin. Earlier she had expressed annoyance with pharmacies because they wouldn't explain policies to their patients. She felt that at times they wouldn't give patients their medication and would say they weren't covered even when they were. She may have been right. For patients who take more than six types of medication and have Medi-Cal,[50] an insurance plan that 40 percent of low-income Californians use, the only way to get all their medicines is to obtain more than a month's supply for at least one of them and then follow up the next month for additional medications. Many patients were unaware that such follow-up might be effective, and it was common to try a different pharmacy because this principle hadn't been explained to them. Fidel had Medi-Cal and she wanted him to realize which medications he should prioritize.

At the end of the visit, Lisa informed Fidel and his wife that she would no longer be at the clinic after that visit and recommended that they see her replacement, Dr. Torres. Lisa knew they would be disappointed and wanted to tell them herself. They were visibly confused and upset, but Lisa assured them that Dr. Torres provided care in the same way she did, as she had trained him. Fidel asked if the new doctor spoke Spanish and if he would be taking patients in the mornings so that he could make such appointments.

Lisa exited the room and walked the patient to the back of the clinic to get someone to check his blood pressure and to make sure that the machine he purchased worked. She asked an intern, a young white woman, to check if the patient's cuff was working. Grateful for the care Lisa had provided Fidel for the last couple of years, Fidel's wife embraced Lisa. *"La quiero mucho doctora. Cuidese."* [I love you so much, doctor. Take care.]

The quality of care that physicians can offer in large HMOs, micro-clinics, and community clinics demonstrates some of the positive outcomes when Latina/o doctors are steered into family and internal medicine, where physicians are sorely needed to provide preventive health to under-resourced Latine communities. A for-profit medical industry, however, places structural limits on the care they would like to provide to all patients that come through their doors. The majority of the Latina/o practitioners I interviewed fused biomedical science with their patients' sociocultural realities, but those working for larger corporatized spaces were limited in the time they could allot to patients and devoted a significant amount of time to re-training other doctors, residents, and colleagues who have absorbed a medical training culture that privileges whiteness. This became a significant source of frustration and burnout.

Mainstream cultural competency training often assumes the culture of the patient is a problem that needs to be understood and a barrier that should be overcome. Cultural competency curriculum is well-intentioned, but it can perpetuate stereotypes and biases. Here we see what happens when that language and cultural barrier falls away, and how Spanish-speaking immigrant patients describe their ailments to co-ethnic doctors. Latine patients recognized the differences when they received language-concordant care from co-ethnic physicians. The practices of Latina/o doctors illustrate how cultural competence encompasses much more than solely Spanish use. While both men and women Latine doctors exhibit varying levels of cultural competency, Latina physicians, in general, possess better skills for practicing cultural humility and make efforts to reduce the power differential.

My observations and interviews indicate that Latina/o physicians practice varying levels of cultural competency, but that structural competency better encompasses the range of issues that patients exhibit during their office visits. Rather than merely treating an injury, ailment, or an organ, most Latina/o physicians I observed recognize the structural forces that limit the care that they can provide as well as how they affect people. While Holmes argues that physicians in the US are not trained to see the social determinants of health problems or to hear these factors when communicated by their patients,[51] most of the Latina/o clinicians I interviewed understand the social determinants of their patients' suffering, and they are severely hampered in the types of treatment they want to offer and what their patients can do. This moral harm is part of the weight that Latina/o doctors carry in a for-profit medical system. Not only do they try to find or scrape together solutions for their patients, but they also expend considerable energy retraining those around them on the importance of understanding their patients' sociocultural and structural realities.

Academic medicine has a professional and ethical responsibility to educate its trainees and health professionals on the history of medicine—including its ugly side—and to critically examine how historical and contemporary political and social factors have created racial/ethnic health disparities.[52] Modeling and instruction should occur with doctors of color and their co-ethnic patients, and with physicians and medical systems in other countries. US medical school curricula can critically unpack the way "race" is used as a proxy marker for the structural roots of health problems such as poverty, and differential access to health care and education. A global comparative lens would also prove useful in the wake of the worldwide COVID-19 crisis, which everyone was exposed to but that disproportionately affected some minority groups.

# 8.

# PREPARING TOMORROW'S *DOCTORES*

IN LATE 2023, two Latina/o physician lawmakers in Congress, Drs. Yadira Caraves and Raul Ruiz, introduced a bipartisan resolution establishing October 1 as the annual National Latino and Latina Physician Day. The resolution aims to recognize Latina/o doctors' contributions to the profession and to bring awareness to the fact that they are only 6 percent of America's doctors in the hope of increasing their representation. The Latina/o doctors whose voices are at the core of this book provide care in a medical context that is a for-profit industry, is predominantly white and heteronormative, has a physician shortage, and has a woeful underrepresentation of Latina/o doctors.[1] This broader context must be considered to adequately address the need, as it influences the white coat's polyvalent weight for men and women who fall under the broad ethnic label of Latinidad.[2]

To put in a larger perspective where Latina/o physicians fall into the political-economic landscape of US health care, I have used an intersectional curious feminist approach as well as an intra-Latine focus. An intersectional curious feminist lens allows us to dissect the interlinked nature of diverse social locations and their connective tissue, and urges us to pay close attention to the range of Latina/o doctors' lives. Latina/o doctors are upwardly mobile and highly skilled, but also wrapped up in larger racial capitalist and masculinized systems beyond their control. I disaggregate Latinidad not to evaluate points of divisions and tensions among Latina/o doctors, but to excavate the particularities of the US case. In placing Latinidad under a microscope and magnifying in-group processes in American medicine, we gain a better view of the intersecting cumulative weights Latina/o physicians inhabit and how these replicate larger patterns of inequality and privilege across various life stages and organizational configurations.

At first glance it appears that Latina/o doctors live charmed lives compared to many of their co-ethnic peers because they make a lot of money and are upwardly socially mobile. However, their experiences are context-contingent as they are stratified across life stages, from gendered dynamics in their families of origin to the educational realm and in their practice. An intra-Latine dynamics lens helps capture our understanding of political-economic advantages and disadvantages among Latinidad, and how Latina/o USMGs have different pathways than positively selected Latin American IMGs. Latin American physicians from other countries were spared US racial categorizations until they set foot in the country as high-status and highly educated immigrants. Subsuming them under the same pan-ethnic and occupational label "Latina/o doctors" without accounting for internal variation erases these distinctions and makes it harder to develop policies that specifically address the circumstances of distinct subgroups. Assessing internal variation suggests most Latina/o USMGs faced roadblocks that international Latin American IMGs did not. Still, physicians trained in Latin America had to complete additional requisites and pay hefty legal fees. The lack of various forms of capital (social, financial, cultural) had grave implications for Latina/o USMGs' entry into medicine, as many of them faced significant structural obstacles when searching for mentors or supportive ethnic networks, which were few and far between.

A main takeaway of my analysis is the critical interlink between gender, ethnicity, and other demographic characteristics and how they shift over time as aspiring Latina/o doctors move up vertically in the medical hierarchy from apprentice to independently licensed practitioners. Latina/o doctors' ethnic capital resources—such as Spanish/English bilingualism and cultural competency—are both valorized and overused to exhaustion within organizations. Ultimately Spanish/English linguistic capital is systematically used as a means to exploit bilingual women in ethnic-based equity tasks, with non-white-presenting and darker-skinned bilingual women having to deplete their ethnic capital resources to a greater degree than their lighter-skinned, monolingual, and/or male colleagues. Latinas experienced repercussions if they did not oblige. To become advocates and better allies for their colleagues who hold the same high-status occupation but are subtly or blatantly overstrained, it behooves all medical professionals to self-reflect and acknowledge the various types of privileges they hold. In many ways, failure to do so would continue to uphold unequal hierarchies and multivalent weights when they benefit from them at the cost of others. Thus, inequality not only stems from a corporatized medical system that requires cultural competency, but also from status biases that patients, nurses, and other doctors exhibit.

This book also expounds on intra-Latine group nuances for those who have gone through medical school and are now part of the medical world that will train future doctors. Future *doctores* that I teach in my "Latin America: Language, Culture and Health" medical school seminar frequently ask: "Why aren't all medical students required to take the courses that we are?" Many of the topics that we covered in that class are addressed in this book. We discuss what health care looks like in other Latin American countries, places where many of them may opt to gain more training. We discuss the important role of Guatemalan Indigenous *iyoms/comadronas* [traditional midwives] who trek across mountains to provide maternal care for little to no compensation and how their local knowledge is devalued in biomedicine. For some students, it was the first time they had ever learned about the inhumane treatment that white American-trained physicians inflicted upon Latines historically. These discussions shape their socialization into medicine, who they want to be as doctors, as well as the systems of oppression and privilege that they will have to learn to navigate in the profession and with a diversity of patients.

These cumulative modes of stratification and privilege are not complete without considering the many patients that physicians care for day after day. This book underscores the need for translators and interpreters who speak multiple languages and are compensated adequately for their labor to create more equitable and inclusive spaces for all physicians and patients. It would also help to reduce the stigma attached to foreign languages. I provide an overview of what doctor-patient interactions can look like when doctors incorporate the socio-cultural and structural realities of the people for whom they take an oath to care. This is important to consider since changing demographic trends in the United States suggest all physicians will be more likely to work with immigrant Latine patients who embody a host of cultural differences. It behooves medical schools to implement programs that train physicians in culturally congruent care and expose them to the structural obstacles that limit their patients from seeking their aid. Failure to do so may continue to encumber physicians of color and inadequately cauterize this incongruence.

The doctors included in this book reflect the diversity of the Latine population in the state of California and identified as Mexican, Central American, South American, Cuban, and Puerto Rican, but none were

Dominican. Socio-demographic characteristics and their observed race matter significantly in their trajectories and workplace experiences. Recent work by sociologist Irene Browne and colleagues suggests that Dominican physicians practicing in Atlanta, Georgia, are of lighter phenotype and attempt to socially distance themselves from working-class and middle-class Mexicans, whom they stereotype as poor and uneducated.[3] Indeed, Dr. Enrique Calderon, a surgeon and one of two Cuban American physicians in my sample, proclaimed that he wanted to retire in Miami, Florida, "where all the good Cubans end up."[4] Although Enrique was born and raised in East Los Angeles, he wanted to return to the thriving Cuban ethnic enclave when he felt ready to hang up his white coat.[5] Latina/o international medical graduates (IMGs) dominate in the Sunshine State; over two-thirds of doctors there trained in Cuba, Nicaragua, Panama, Venezuela, or the Dominican Republic.[6] This book brings to the forefront the experiences of Latina/o doctors who made their successful careers in California and who, like Enrique, are mostly USMGs with a much different demographic composition than physicians in the peninsular southeastern state. Latina/o physicians working in other states or countries may have different experiences from those I have recounted here. Given that Florida and Texas have a higher percentage of Latina/o doctors, future research should capture how a for-profit medical industry operates in states that have distinct regional racial hierarchies by being attuned to differences between USMG and IMG experiences, with a particular focus on gendered processes.

Gendered processes will be critical to maintain as a mode of inquiry as American medicine is changing to include more women than ever, and more Latinas are applying to medicine over their male counterparts; currently, Latinas make up 55.3 percent of Latine applicants to medical school. In 2019, the overall percentage of women applicants was 50.9 percent.[7] The United States has only 2.6 physicians per 1,000 people. This puts it behind sixty countries in the world.[8] Cuba, on the other hand, has the highest doctor-to-patient ratio in the world (8.4 per

1,000), with more than three times the coverage of the United States. It also has a more feminized conception of "physicianhood," as the majority of its doctors are women. We can use the case of Cuba to extrapolate what a potential future feminized medical workforce might mean for doctors who practice in America.

## MEDICINE IN CUBA AS A COUNTERPOINT

In January 2020, I took a research trip to Cuba with the UC-Cuba Academic Initiative, a multicampus network of scholars, to explore how another country has produced a feminized workforce in medicine despite the many embargoes and restrictions imposed upon it. Speaking with a Cuban doctor I met sheds light on what future policymakers might consider.

One early Friday morning in January 2020, a *Cuber*—Cuban Uber—picked me up from the UC-Cuba sponsors' middle-class neighborhood near *La Habana*. The driver was set to take me to the hospital where Emma, a Cuban biochemist and UC-Cuba mentor and support person in Havana, worked. Emma was a key informant, and when I explained the purpose of my visit, she jokingly said that there were more women biochemists and doctors than men in Cuba. I quickly came to learn that nearly 62 percent of physicians in Cuba are women and they are concentrated in specialties like neonatology or pediatrics.[9] It was common to come across women in various STEM fields in Cuba, a striking experience after seeing the small numbers of women of color doctors and in STEM overall in the United States. *The Weight of the White Coat* excavates why the numbers in the US are so low; I was there to learn something about why this is not the case in Cuba.

As soon as the taxi driver dropped me off Emma handed me a white coat to put on while she gave him parking instructions. *"Ten, ponte esta bata*" [Here, put this coat on], she said. As I slipped it over my arms, the glee that newly admitted medical students must feel at their white coat ceremonies rushed through my body. We made our way into the building and walked up the stairs into one of the lobbies, where several patients were waiting. I later learned that many of them were internal migrants from Santiago de Cuba, a southeastern area of the island. We made our way to the right, down a small corridor to the neonatal lab. Emma worked in this lab and her primary job was retrieving blood samples from infants and their mothers after they were born to gather genetic information. Most of the supplies in their small office were donated by UC-Cuba affiliates, such as pre-inked rubber stamps for forms and a backup generator so they would not lose patient files when the power went out. Emma noted the scarcity of resources in the hospital and the island: *"No tenemos nada. Ni bolígrafo, ni papel. Nada."* [We don't have anything. No pens, or paper. Nothing].[10] The effects of the economic embargo, sanctions, and the collapse of the Soviet Union, the island's previous main diplomatic and economic source, were clear.

Emma had set up a meeting for me with a Cuban woman neonatologist who worked in her same unit, Dr. Arianny Mirabal.[11] A *Cubana blanca,* a white woman, Arianny (as she told me to call her) was wearing purple-rimmed glasses, blue pants, and her white coat. She had dyed blond hair in a disheveled updo. I followed the same interview protocol with Arianny that I did with physicians in California and asked her about her family, the dynamics of her job, and her relationships with her coworkers and patients. Arianny put on a thirty-minute timer (another donation from UC-Cuba) for our interview. She sat at her small desk and filled out some paperwork as I asked her questions. She explained that her siblings (two women, one man) were now living in Miami, Florida, in the thriving Cuban enclave. Unlike Enrique's parents, who fled the island after the Cuban Revolution in 1959, her parents remained in Cuba. Her mother worked at a Cuban university as a translator and her father was an electrician; both were ecstatic that she was a doctor. Arianny presented an interesting case of a middle-class family that remained on the island rather than following the Golden Exiles, the first wave of Cuban refugees post-1959, and those who made their way later like her siblings. As the responsible eldest daughter, Arianny had helped her siblings get to Miami via Mexico. All of them were professionals (teacher, pharmacist) or learned a trade (mechanic). To attain initial visas and then passports for all her siblings to move cost her *"un montón de dinero"* [a lot of money] in ways that echo the migration patterns of high-skilled Latin American IMGs. She seemed perturbed.

Unlike USMG Latina/o physicians who amassed six-figure loans, Arianny explained that going to school in Cuba had not cost her a dime, a common circumstance in other countries. Medical education in Cuba is provided free to people from communities with poor access to health care on condition that upon graduation they return to serve them. *"Aquí no cuesta nada. Se estudia y se supera. Afortunadamente eso no ha cambiado. Es la oportunidad de estudiar y no tener que pagarlo. Es una barbaridad lo que se tiene que pagar."* [Here it doesn't cost anything. You can study and prevail. Fortunately, that hasn't changed. It is the opportunity to study and not have to pay for it. It is a barbarity what people must pay.] When I asked her why she thought there were so many women doctors in Cuba, she said, *"Las cubanas tenemos la oportunidad de estudiar. Somos mas lanzadas."* [Cuban women have the opportunity to study. We are more daring.]

Arianny's words help us glean some insight into how another country has managed to produce so many women scientists. Her words highlight that financial strain was not a major constraint for her, and neither was the weaker K-9 preparation that many poorer and first-generation Latina/o physicians told me about in contrast to IMGs who had completed their schooling in Latin America with mostly co-ethnic peers. Arianny and her parents paid to send her siblings to the United States where they could re-establish their careers, a feat made possible due to the provisions of the Cuban Adjustment Act of 1966, which remains in effect today. Mexican and Central American-origin physicians trained in US schools and those who had college-educated parents in the home country who could not recertify their degrees in the US rarely had these advantages.

The experiences of Latin American IMGs who were still trying to learn where they fell in US racial strata and what US racism looked like had led me to expect that Arianny would be just as innocent. Indeed, as a *Cubana blanca*, Arianny did not notice any racial microaggressions or disrespect in her career. She described her coworkers as *"bién chéveres"* [cool] and said of her patients, *"Los pacientes no intentan avasallaste. Tú eres la solución para su problema. Ellos están en tus manos."* [The patients don't try to run you over. You are the solution to their problem. They are in your hands.] White racial privilege garnered her respect from patients in ways similar to bilingual white-presenting Latino doctors in America.

Arianny also reflected on this. She referenced the distinct racial dynamics in Cuba when I asked about the racial composition of doctors to explain that skin color was not a deterrent to access to higher education. *"Eso no esta muy marcado. Somos mezcla. No somos 100% puro. Hay mucha diversidad."* [That (race) is not as marked. We are a mix. We are not one hundred percent pure. There is a lot of diversity.] Indeed, walking down the street, and in the doctor's office, I saw many Cubans of various hues. She explained that, unlike the US which has a rigid Black-white binary, distinctions on the island were made by region. Her patients were also primarily co-ethnics from either Havana or Santiago de Cuba. She gave me the example of one of her patients who had just given birth: *"Esta madre dio luz aquí. Yo recibí el parto. Se nota la diferencia del acento. En seguida notas un Habanero y un Santiaguero. En La Habana hay mucha población de Santiago. Y se notan las diferencias en la manera de hablar, en la provincia, en los vocabolos. Por ejemplo en La Habana decimos platanito y ellos dicen guineo. Es lo mismo."* [This mother gave birth here. I delivered the baby. You can notice the difference in the accent. You can quickly notice the difference between someone from Havana and Santiago. In Havana, there is a large number of people from Santiago. You can notice the difference quickly in their ways of speaking, the province, and the vocabulary. For example, in Havana we say *banana* and they say *guineo*. It is the same.]

Naturally, Arianny's interpretations of race relations on the island heavily contrasted with Emma's. Emma was of a far darker hue and from a poorer family than Arianny. She told me that in Cuba she would be classified as a *Cubana negra* or *morena*.[12] As a lab technician, Emma was also at the bottom of the medical hierarchy.

Emma had engaged in medical missions to provide care to people in other countries, and her status as a lab technician influenced the locations she was sent to for these medical exchange missions. She had engaged in these medical missions to attain resources for her mother, as medical professionals who participate can ship *electrodomésticos* such as refrigerators or washing machines to Cuba for free. Arianny had never done this. She likely had some political "pull" that kept her from traveling abroad and providing care in slums and the most marginalized rural communities, whereas Emma felt conscripted to do so.

While Emma was not a medical doctor, she regularly signed up for these missions, as medical diplomacy is the island's most lucrative export activity.[13] Emma had gone to Chitato, Angola, and Venezuela to provide care to mothers and their infants in the most underserved areas. Some Cuban medical doctors travel to other countries like Italy, Chile, Venezuela, Liberia, Mozambique, Pakistan, or Mexico in times of national crises, like the worldwide pandemic or when large groups of migrants arrive at the US-Mexico border. Cuba even offered to send the Bush administration up to 1,000 doctors trained in disaster relief after Hurricane Katrina, which the US rejected.[14] Medical diplomacy also means that doctors and scientists are sent to other countries often, sometimes creating a type of "brain drain" in Cuba even though there is an oversupply of physicians.

A study that focuses on Cuban doctors who engage in medical diplomacy missions could be quite illuminating, as these medical missions gave Emma a comparative understanding of race that she then brought back to Cuba. Emma felt that Angolans treated her well and respected her expertise and assessments. *"Todos los angolos me trataban muy bién. No hay ni un angolo que me trato mal. El problema son los cubanos. Y te digo son los cubanos a todos niveles, de los marginados y los del centro Habana."* [All of the Angolans treated me well. There wasn't one Angolan that treated me poorly. The problem is Cubans. And I will tell you it is Cubans at all levels, from marginalized areas to the city center.] El Centro was a dense community with poorer Cubans of all shades and hues. In contrast to Arianny, Emma felt that while the revolution in the late 1950s had attempted to eliminate discrimination and gave the perception that it did, it had other consequences for her as a highly educated *Cubana negra* in a career that was mostly held by other women. *"Hay diferentes manifestaciones de discriminación"* [There are different manifestations of discrimination], she said. While she had not experienced gender discrimination, she had faced status discrimination. Racial capitalism manifested differently for medical personnel on the island.

I use these field notes to contrast how skin tone and gender produce different weights of oppression or advantage for physicians, especially when we examine in-group dynamics domestically and globally. The fieldnotes I captured during my stay bolster my argument of the white coat's polyvalence because they cast additional light on how gender, racism, and colorism intersected for Latinas/os in US medicine and therefore their context-contingent plasticity.

American medical institutions can begin to address and mend many of the hierarchies I describe. I find that demonstrations of gendered deference matter for retention rates among Latina doctors. Examining cultural understandings of gendered deference and demeanor provides a next-generation framework to create higher education institutions that reflect the population institutions seek to recruit and intend to serve. Medical organizations should not only deem bilingualism an asset among apprentices, staff, or medical students, but should also offer higher compensation for possessing this skill by working a stipend into salaries to remunerate them appropriately for performing this critical labor that saves lives. Because the data reveal that Latina physicians are disproportionately performing this shadow labor, the compensation should account for the average number of patients they see in which doctors must use their linguistic capital to provide care. They can also be provided with multilingual staff. Failure to implement formal policies that address gendered deference in medicine could potentially serve as a deterrent and continue pushing Latinas to exit STEM at multiple points in their trajectories. Doctors begin to get socialized into the profession as medical students and are exposed to a host of cultural, gendered, and racialized biases early on. Many of these biases are imbued with stereotypical cultural elements or status beliefs about gender, and Latina/o doctors spend a considerable amount of time navigating, disrupting, or resigning themselves to them daily. Creating formal rules that describe lack of gendered deference as noncollegial behavior in the workplace would protect not only Latina physicians but all medical workers and patients. Ultimately a better workplace for all will serve patient outcomes and is essential for a country where, given the aging of the population, the need for structurally competent medical care will certainly grow.

# AFTERWORD

Doctoring during and after COVID-19

░░░░░░░░░░░░░░░░░░░░░░░░░░░░░░░░░░░░░░░░░░░░░░░░░░░░░░░░░░░░░░░░░░░░░░░░░░░░░░░░░░░░░░░░░░░

DR. MARISA DELGADO was the only Latina pathologist in her unit when I interviewed her in March 2020. Marisa, of course, was early to recognize the need for what was called at the time social distancing, and the interview took place over Zoom. Just a week before we talked, she had completed an autopsy on a COVID-19-positive patient. Marisa did not know that this patient had succumbed to the illness until she determined the cause of death, and she was self-quarantining before returning to work and interacting with other patients and coworkers again. Assessing Latina/o physicians' experiences during the pandemic was not a primary focus of my analysis, but Marisa and the other doctors I spoke to during this period and after had many tales to tell of being cultural brokers—intermediaries between patients and

Portions of this afterword are related to a previously published article: Flores, Glenda M. 2020. "Latina Physicians as 'Essential' Workers." *Contexts* 19(4): 62–64.

others—on the front lines. Marisa was one of the few pathologists treating people of color in a Los Angeles hospital that received many "overflow" patients, what uninsured and indigent patients were called. They were mostly poor African Americans and Latinos/as. In the time of COVID-19, cultural competencies were tested for Latina/o doctors who treated both co-ethnic and non-Latine essential workers who were disproportionately affected by the virus.

The pandemic elicited childhood memories of trauma for Marisa. Her parents, a schoolteacher and civil engineer, fled Nicaragua for America when she was five years old, fearing for their lives and hers. Growing up with other Nicaraguan immigrants in San Francisco, she was accustomed to hearing brutal "war zone" stories from Central America. She assessed the global health crisis occurring in 2020 through this dual frame of reference lens, suggesting that inequities fade when people are suffering because patients do not care who provides them with aid, and doctors treat whoever is in front of them without cultural biases. At the onset of the novel coronavirus pandemic, Marisa felt that everyone in her county hospital jumped in and triaged the situation without taking note of doctors' or patients' social location or demographics. All hierarchies seemed to vanish. It was an all-hands-on-deck approach to staffing and included anyone who possessed the right scrubs, mask, and stethoscope. This perspective was short-lived.

Others were emphatic that the pandemic only exacerbated and magnified existing cracks and inequities in health care, pushing everyone to the breaking point. This was Marisa's experience as well, to some degree. Because she was the only Spanish speaker in her specialty in the facility, coworkers often called on Marisa to explain their results and treatment procedures to patients in a language they understood. In the time of COVID-19, Latina/o physicians working and treating patients in less-resourced communities were crucial to providing culturally competent care and helping numerous patients understand the public health implications of the virus in ways they could comprehend.

This often meant relaying grim news to a patient's loved ones over the phone. The experiences of Latina/o doctors on the front lines of the pandemic that disproportionately affected co-ethnic communities amplified the weight of the white coat, especially for Spanish/English bilingual women. Much of their work remained unacknowledged and performing this labor took a toll.

Despite limited numbers, Latina/o doctors were vital for understanding the spread of COVID-19. In December 2020, Dr. Susan López wrote in the *HuffPost*, "I have never taken care of more Spanish speakers, undocumented patients, Latinx patients or Black patients than I have during the pandemic." In her piece, Dr. López, who practices internal medicine, noted that treating so many co-ethnics had taken a toll on her well-being. She felt that the unclear messaging many Spanish-speaking communities received missed specific structural and cultural issues. As a Mexican American physician, she was conscious that many Latine workers were front-line "essential" workers who could not stay at home. Many lived in multigenerational homes and could not be isolated from the most vulnerable.

Benito, another doctor I interviewed over Zoom in the early months of the pandemic, explained that he engaged in community forums where he would broadcast information in Spanish to immigrant communities. He became one of the main physicians that news and media outlets would regularly seek to answer common questions regarding the vaccine. He addressed questions that callers had about *remedios caseros* [home remedies] they had heard would stave off the virus, or that they used to allay their symptoms. Such physicians were indispensable to these communities for their culturally competent care and possessed crucial skills that are often uncompensated, tokenized, and taken for granted, even by themselves at times. They were what I call "racialized tokens" because they experienced a series of uncomfortable situations and performed additional shadow labor—important unrecognized tasks—when they were numerical minorities in white-collar occupations. Benito still engages in this work today and is an active figure in ethnic medical programs that train future doctors. Like many others, he draws from his experiences during the pandemic to train future Latine doctors on the importance of taking a structurally competent lens when assessing health patterns among disenfranchised patients.

While Latina/o physicians stepped up to the plate to serve co-ethnic communities, the novel coronavirus demonstrated that providing culturally competent care also came at a cost. Dr. Lizet Ramos worked in emergency medicine in an underserved hospital, and she spoke with me over Zoom in May 2020. She presented as a light-skinned Latina, and pre-COVID-19 she could pass, reducing the likelihood of racial discrimination at work. However, Lizet had a very slight accent indicative of a native Spanish speaker that sometimes gave her away, and medical protective garb seemed to increase patients' response to that accent in the absence of other information. She said, "You're wearing the gown, face mask and goggles. No one can see your ID. . . . My badge has a big red thing that says doctor on it. Sometimes [patients] think you're the nurse and say, 'I want to speak to the doctor.' I say, 'You've been speaking to her for 30 minutes.'" While Lizet felt she was culturally competent to aid patients of various social and economic backgrounds, she understood her ethnicity and gender meant that patients did not fully recognize her medical expertise, favoring medical providers who conformed to the conventional white male norm of high-status occupations. She felt the pandemic compounded inequities for Spanish/English bilingual doctors.

While culturally competent care is critical to working with marginalized communities, it is often undervalued and undermined by institutions and colleagues, especially for bilingual women. Dr. Estrella Llanos, a Mexican/Puerto Rican heritage doctor, explained that pharmaceutical companies reached out to her about clinical trials for the COVID-19 vaccine for children, but someone in a leadership capacity at her institution got "really upset" that they approached her instead of him. His hostile actions were on the verge of a Title IX (gender discrimination) violation, and their employer required him to undergo counseling. Reflecting on the incident, Estrella protested that if "she was a man" she would have been allotted the flexibility to engage in clinical work. Her important contributions to these interventions—which were crucial to protecting all children—were minimized and challenged because she was Latina.

COVID-19 was a brutally isolating disease. The culturally competent care Latina/o physicians provided on the job was critical to supporting their co-ethnic patients and their family members who could not physically be there with them. Yet it took a hefty toll, especially on women, who continued to be burdened more than men by interpretation demands. Both Latina/o physicians explained their Spanish/English linguistic and bicultural skills were an ethnic asset in their jobs, but using them to facilitate others' clinical interactions was quite different from using them to facilitate their own. Estrella strongly valued the linguistic and cultural competence that made the health community fairs she ran in predominantly Mexican and Central American immigrant cities like Santa Ana effective and the improved care she could provide hospitalized Spanish speakers. However, she explained that white doctors relied on her uncompensated bilingual labor to explain to every Spanish-speaking patient what was going on with their health despite the fact it was not her job to do so.

During the global pandemic, the linguistic and cultural resources Latina/o clinicians provided for their patients, coworkers, and the medical profession as a whole were all the more indispensable. Yet much as they had been before, their efforts were often invisibilized, even though patients and their families requested and desperately wished for them. The novel coronavirus put these doctors, who already felt the weight on their shoulders, to the test, and the pre-existing cracks in American health care became faults. So long as Latina/o doctors work in the "token" context, so long as they are systematically asked to execute tasks that others performing the same job can out-source, they will be extremely vulnerable to burnout. Making struc-tural change at every level is vital if we are to take care of the populace during abnormal times, and to begin the process of inoculating our-selves during normal times.

# Physicians' Demographic Statistics by Sex ($N = 74$)

Physicians' Demographic Statistics by Sex ($N = 74$)

| Characteristics | Female Physicians | Male Physicians | Total/ Percent |
|---|---|---|---|
| **Generational Level** | | | |
| 1st | 7 (18%) | 3 (9%) | 10 (13%) |
| 1.5 | 10 (26%) | 3 (9%) | 13 (18%) |
| 2nd | 11 (28%) | 26 (74%) | 37 (**50%**) |
| 3rd+ | 8 (20%) | 2 (6%) | 10 (14%) |
| Other[a] | 3 (8%) | 1 (3%) | 4 (5%) |
| **Ethnicity** | | | |
| Mexican[b] | 23 (**59%**) | 27 (**77%**) | 50 (**68%**) |
| Central American | 4 (12%) | 1 (3%) | 5 (7%) |
| South American | 8 (21%) | 5 (14%) | 13 (**18%**) |
| Caribbean | 4 (8%) | 2 (6%) | 6 (7%) |
| **Medical School** | | | |
| USMG | 32 (82%) | 31 (89%) | 63 (85%) |
| IMG | 7 (18%) | 4 (11%) | 11 (15%) |
| **Language** | | | |
| Monolingual (English only) | 2 (6%) | 1 (3%) | 3 (4%) |
| Bilingual (English and Spanish) | 37 (95%) | 34 (97%) | 71 (96%) |
| **Age (years)** | | | |
| 29–40 | 16 (41%) | 22 (63%) | 38 (53%) |
| 41–60 | 17 (44%) | 11 (31%) | 28 (36%) |
| ≥60 | 6 (15%) | 2 (6%) | 8 (11%) |
| **Years Practicing** | | | |
| 0–10 | 18 (46%) | 22 (63%) | 40 (55%) |
| 11–20 | 9 (23%) | 8 (23%) | 17 (23%) |
| 21–30 | 7 (18%) | 3 (9%) | 10 (12%) |
| ≥31 | 5 (13%) | 2 (6%) | 7 (10%) |
| **Specialty** | | | |
| Family Medicine | 12 (**31%**) | 8 (23%) | 20 (**27%**) |
| Internal Medicine | 6 (15%) | 11 (**31%**) | 17 (**23%**) |
| Pediatrics | 6 (15%) | 2 (6%) | 8 (11%) |
| OBGYN | 2 (5%) | - | 2 (3%) |
| Surgery | 2 (5%) | 9 (26%) | 11 (15%) |
| Other[c] | 11 (28%) | 5 (14%) | 16 (21%) |
| **Annual Income (US$)[d]** | | | |
| 40,000–100,000 | 5 (13%) | 4 (11%) | 9 (12%) |
| 100,001–200,000 | 13 (33%) | 7 (20%) | 20 (27%) |

| | | | |
|---|---|---|---|
| 200,001–300,000 | 11 (28%) | 11 (31%) | 22 (30%) |
| ≥300,001 | 6 (15%) | 12 (34%) | 18 (24%) |
| Not Reported | 4 (10%) | 1 (3%) | 5 (7%) |
| **Marital Status** | | | |
| Single | 13 (33%) | 11 (31%) | 24 (32%) |
| Married | 25 (64%) | 22 (63%) | 47 (64%) |
| Divorced | 1 (3%) | 2 (6%) | 3 (4%) |
| n (%) | 39 (53%) | 35 (47%) | 74 (100%) |

[a] "Other" includes three Puerto Rican women participants, two of whom studied in Puerto Rico.

[b] This category consists of participants who self-identified as Mexican, Mexican American, Chicana/o, Xicano and one Mexican/Puerto Rican respondent.

[c] "Other specialty" category includes ophthalmology, rheumatology, dermatology, gastroenterology, pathology, osteopathy, podiatry, psychiatry, neurology, and cardiology.

[d] Four female and one male participant did not provide annual income.

# Latine Medical Students' Demographics ($N = 12$)

Latine Medical Students' Demographics ($N = 12$)

| Pseudonym | Generation | Age | Race/Ethnicity | Parent (POB) | Undergraduate Major | Medical School Year |
|---|---|---|---|---|---|---|
| Jason | 1.5 | 25 | Latino | Peru | Human Biology | 1st |
| Jennifer | 1.5 | 25 | Mexican | Mexico | Human Biology | 2nd |
| Alex | 2nd | 25 | Mexican American | Mexico | Biology | 2nd |
| Camelia | 2nd | 26 | Latina | Mexico | Biology | 3rd |
| Eddie | 2nd | 28 | Latino | El Salvador | Molecular Biology | 4th |
| Jasmine | 2nd | 25 | Mexican | Mexico | Biology | 2nd |
| Javier | 2nd | 24 | Chilean | Chile | Biochemistry | 2nd |
| Maritza | 2nd | 25 | Hondureña/Salvadoreña | Central America | Social Welfare and Education | 1st |
| Pamela | 2nd | 24 | Latino | El Salvador / Mexico | Anthropology | 2nd |
| Rubén | 2nd | 25 | Latino | El Salvador / Israel | Biological Sciences | 2nd |
| Sylvia | 2nd | 24 | Latina | Peru | Biology | 1st |
| Irene | 2nd | 29 | Mexican | Mexico | Biological Sciences | 2nd |

# Notes

1. The children of Latine immigrants, who are skilled in two vernaculars, often serve as language and cultural brokers for their parents. Not only do they engage in social responsibilities such as driving parents to doctors' appointments or make important phone calls when dealing with bureaucratic officials (Vallejo 2012), but they also shoulder basic and more complicated verbal exchanges for their non-English speaking parents and relatives in various institutional realms (see Estrada 2019; Kwon 2015; Delgado 2020; Orellana 2009; Valenzuela 1999).

2. Hispanic female physicians tend to be young, with a median age of forty. A few are older than sixty-five. Nearly 70 percent of all Hispanic female physicians speak Spanish at home (Anaya et al. 2022; Anaya et al. 2023).

3. Although the term "Latinx" has gained prominence and is used to disrupt the gender binary in the United States, none of the physicians included in the study used the term to self-identify. Some physicians were born in Latin America and were unfamiliar

with the term. For this reason, I use "Latina/o," a panethnic label that denotes the diasporic nature of the sample when referring to respondents. I use "Latine" when referring to the entire population because the plural form of doctors in the Spanish language is inclusive: *doctores*.

4. AAMC 2022.

5. See the work of Collins 2019; Crenshaw 1991; and Enloe 2004.

6. For more on international medical graduates see Jenkins 2021 and Yrigoyen and Zambrana 1979.

7. For more on intersectionalities in organizations see Hulko 2009 and Holvino 2010.

8. For other studies that use an intersectionalities framework among, and within, Latinidad see Zinn and Zambrana 2019; Lugo-Lugo 2008; and Falcón 2008.

9. AAMC 2014.

10. For more on the racial/ethnic composition of primary care physicians see Xierali and Nivet 2018.

11. Basu et al., 2019.

12. Abel Valenzuela (1999) demonstrates that Mexican-origin girls, more so than boys, served as tutors or interpreters and participated in activities that required detailed explanations, mediated difficult transactions, or had greater responsibility when helping their parents and younger siblings settle in the United States. Boys, despite their involvement in household activities, did not have the same responsibilities as girls did unless they were the eldest child. Emir Estrada and Pierrette Hondagneu-Sotelo (2013) also write about these gendered dynamics among the children of street vendors.

13. Gender plays an important role on who shoulders most of this interpretation work in both private and public spheres (see Lee and Hatteberg 2015; López 2002; Estrada 2019; Valenzuela 1999; Smith 2005; Flores and Bañuelos 2021; Flores 2020b). These bilingual skills are often enhanced and reinforced for girls who face greater constraints in their homes while boys are given more physical freedom outside of the household and access to public spaces (see Smith 2005; López 2002; Ovink 2013; Estrada 2019).

14. See Brenda Beagan's (2001) study of quotidian inequities related to the intersection of race, gender, class, and sexuality in the lives of men and women physicians in Canada. While Canada is presumed to be a racial mosaic, Beagan

contends that women worried about their body shape, hair, and make-up. Moreover, LGBTQ+ individuals felt pressured to hide their identities.

15. For more see Molina 2006.

16. Molina 2011.

17. A. García 1982; Espino and Tajima-Peña 2016; and Gutiérrez 2008 all discuss fertility and Latina immigrants in greater detail in their works.

18. This practice also happened to Native American women living in reservations. Historian Brianna Theobald (2019) explains that in the 1970s physicians sterilized between 25 and 42 percent of Native women of childbearing age. Some of these procedures occurred in government-operated hospitals. Women of All Red Nations (WARN) explained that physicians performed these procedures coercively and with genocidal intentions.

19. The stethoscope or the black bag also personifies or symbolizes physicianhood.

20. White-coat ceremonies are a recent phenomenon that began in the late 1980s and early 1990s. Before medicine became a scientific enterprise, it was customary for doctors to wear black garb. Michel Foucault's *The Birth of the Clinic* (1994) gives an overview of the medical gaze and medical school cultures. He chronicles how medical knowledge and diagnoses changed from religious interpretations of ailments to verifiable observations of the body.

21. Brewer and colleagues (2020) show how gender inequality is perpetuated in emergency medical education, when women are evaluated more harshly as they transition from student to professional and colleague roles.

22. For more on racial capitalism in health care see Pirtle 2020.

23. The medical profession has changed in the last several decades. Once it was common for doctors (who were mostly white men) to have their own practice. Today, the reverse is true, where most doctors (white or not) do not have their own practice and work for large organizations.

24. Lombarts and Verghese 2022.

25. Asians are dwarfed by whites; they represent 21 percent of the active doctor population (American Association of Medical Colleges 2022).

26. Anaya et al. 2023.

27. Goshua 2019, quote from 36; Lorber 1984. Also see Romano (2018) for an assessment of how white privilege manifested for him as a white male physician in training.

28. Cassell 1997, quote from 50.

29. *Dr. 90210*, a reality series that ran in 2004–2008 and focused on cosmetic surgeries in the wealthy suburb of Beverly Hills, California, depicted several Latino doctors such as Robert Rey.

30. Women were barred until 1876, when the first "qualified" woman physician inducted into the association was white American physician Dr. Sarah Hackett Stevenson. Black doctors formed their own medical society, the National Medical Association (NMA), in 1895. See Dan Ly's (2022) work for a historical overview of Black physicians' representation and incomes.

31. Martinez et al., 2019; AAMC 2022b. California, Florida, and Texas are followed by Puerto Rico. New York and Illinois rank fourth and fifth among US states.

32. Anaya et al. 2023; AAMC 2022a.

33. Double jeopardy is used to indicate the intersection of race and gender, while triple oppression emphasizes the interlinked nature of race, gender, and class. For more on the simultaneity perspective in organization studies see Holvino 2010.

34. Flores 2017.

35. Garcia-López and Segura 2008; Chávez 2011, 2019.

36. Gándara 1995.

37. Grijalva and Coombs 1997.

38. Krogstad and Gonzalez-Barrera 2015.

39. Ochoa 2004.

40. F. Padilla 1985; Oboler 1995; Ochoa 2004; Mallet and Pinto-Coelho 2018; Osuna 2015.

41. Zinn and Zambrana 2019; Lugo-Lugo 2008.

42. Espiritu 1993, 14.

43. Tiako et al. 2021; Geiger et al. 2024.

44. Talamantes et al. 2016; Talamantes et al. 2019.

45. Only one IMG doctor in my sample was a US citizen (born in Chula Vista) and opted to pursue his medical education across the border in Mexico.

46. The first efforts to modulate the influx of foreign-trained doctors occurred in 1938 when the AMA required all international medical graduates (IMGs) to obtain US citizenship prior to being licensed.

47. They must have Educational Commission for Foreign Medical Graduates (ECFMG) certification, pass the United States Medical Licensing Examination

(USMLE) Step 1, Step 2 clinical knowledge, Step 2 clinical skills (these must be completed regardless to obtain ECFMG certification), and Step 3, and obtain a state medical license.

48. In 1948 the Smith-Mundt Act was developed to allow for extended exchange visitor (J) visas to IMGs for the first time. This allowed foreign-trained doctors to pursue postgraduate training in the US. Those interested in practicing in the United States had to return to their home country after residency for at least two years prior to applying for reentry or legal permanent residency in the US, which, upon being granted, would allow them to practice medicine in the United States.

49. The Conrad 30 waiver program allows J-1 international medical graduates (IMGs) to apply for a waiver of the 2-year foreign residence requirement upon completion of the J-1 exchange visitor program.

50. Latinas/os are also underrepresented in the nursing occupation (see Vogt and Taningco 2008).

51. Monk 2021.

52. Murguia and Telles 1996; Kim and Calzada 2019.

53. Uzogara 2019.

54. Roth 2016; Maghbouleh 2017.

55. Dixon and Telles 2017.

56. Acker 2006; Tiako et al. 2021; Ray 2019.

57. Ray 2019.

58. Wingfield and Alston 2014, 276.

59. Acker 2006.

60. Ong 2005, 598.

61. Kwon and Adams 2018.

62. Molina et al. 2020, 387; Zelek and Phillips 2003.

63. Bhatt 2013.

64. Wingfield and Chávez 2020.

65. Wingfield 2019.

66. Zinn 2001.

67. McCall 2005, 1787.

68. Ahn et al., 2022; Olivares-Urueta 2012.

69. In January 2020, Raul Fernández and I traveled to Cuba when there were initial murmurs that the novel coronavirus existed. During this time

the main precaution we were given was to wash our hands for twenty seconds.

70. I had originally planned to do this program in October 2020 but was unable to participate until October 2022.

71. My teacher informed me that my Spanish was more advanced compared to the majority of other students at the institute who were learning the language. Yet, while I was able to hold a conversation, I immediately learned that medical Spanish required learning many more adjectives associated with medical terminology related to specialties and general patient descriptors.

72. Crenshaw 1991; Solórzano and Yosso 2002.

CHAPTER 2

1. See Tina Vasquez, "A Chat with Sandra Cisneros, Beloved Author & Patron Saint of Chingonas," October 7, 2015, https://themuse.jezebel.com/a-chat-with-sandra-cisneros-beloved-author-patron-sa-1734661762.

2. While Latina physicians noted that patriarchy was an element of Latin American societies, patriarchy exists in the US context as well.

3. Chávez 2019.

4. Some of the Latina physicians I interviewed referred to Dr. Calliope Torres of the hit television series *Grey's Anatomy* as a point of identification. "Callie's" character is a US medical graduate (USMG) whose wealthy Cuban father funded her entire higher educational journey. She specialized in orthopedic surgery and usually clashed with her father over her career choice and sexuality as a member of the LGBTQ+ community.

5. Hondagneu-Sotelo (1994) explains that women's entry into the low-wage sectors in the US and access to public spaces created more egalitarian relationships. In *Family Secrets,* Gloria González-López (2005) explains the troubling, gendered ideologies of familial incest towards Mexican daughters in Mexico by fathers and sons. Also see Zinn 1979 and Fernandez-Kelly and Garcia 1997.

6. Cabrera, Flores, and Reich 2024.

7. Vasquez-Tokos (2011) focused mostly on Mexican heritage families. However, Dr. Carolina Baez, a Puerto Rican physician trained on the island, also mentioned how her very religious mother responded to her rigorous study habits on the weekends. Carolina mentioned, "For my mom, it was like sacrilege to

not stay at home on Sundays and go to church, and help out family." Both of her parents were very proud of her career choice, but she primarily received messages about familial obligations from her mother.

8. Zambrana and Hurtado 2015.

9. The overwhelming majority of the Caribbean respondents (West Indian, Dominican, or Haitian) in López's 2005 study were racialized as Black and were raised by mothers who worked in low-wage sectors in New York. Some mothers were undocumented. Interestingly, four of the five Caribbean-heritage women physicians (Puerto Rican or Cuban) in my sample were raised by at least one parent who had a college degree. Except for Dr. Soraida Ocasio (see chapter 6) they were lighter-skinned. All of them possessed U.S. citizenship status.

10. Benito was offered the scholarship because he was earning a high school diploma at Don Bosco Technical School's Architecture and Construction Engineering technology program.

11. Many Salvadorans of various class backgrounds were blacklisted as enemies of the Salvadoran government and feared that their loved ones would be jailed or disappeared at the hands of death squads.

12. For more on the downward mobility experiences of immigrant Latines who are professionals in their country of origin see the work of Daniel Dohan (2003) and Cecilia Ménjivar (2000).

13. Gloria's father was a journalist and her mother a psychologist in Argentina.

14. Enrique's wife was a white woman who worked as a physician's assistant.

15. Familism or *familismo* has been used to describe close-knit ties among some working-class immigrant Latino families; however, Ovink (2013) incorporates a gendered element to this concept.

16. Chávez 2019.

17. Kibria 1993; Cabrera, Flores, and Reich, 2024.

18. Dasgupta and DasGupta 1996. For more on gendered dynamics in immigrant families of color see the work of Mary Waters (1996) and Diane Wolf (1997).

19. Ovink 2013, 275.

20. López 2002.

21. Chapter 4 delves deeper into the explanations doctors give for working in marginalized or affluent communities and the messages they receive from mentors, professors, and coworkers.

22. Gónzalez-López 2004.

23. Vasquez 2001.

24. Bettie 2003; Zambrana and Hurtado 2015; Flores 2017.

25. Smith 2005.

26. For an analysis of how college-educated Latinas are more likely than sons to be regarded as a new resource for lifting family fortunes, see Ovink 2013.

27. The California College Promise Grant is available for students planning to or currently attending a California community college and waives per-unit tuition fees. To be eligible for the grant students must demonstrate financial need, be a resident of California, and be planning to or currently attending a community college. Recipients must maintain a 2.0 grade point average.

28. González-López 2004.

29. See Raffaelli and Green 2003; L. Garcia 2012; Parra and Garcia 2023.

30. The literal English translation of this idiom is "do not come out with your Sunday seven." In Mexican and Central American parlance, this is a general warning not to do something foolish, but when directed to unmarried women generally refers to an unplanned pregnancy.

31. See Zhou and Bankston (1998) for an examination of the contradictory family dynamics and unfair gendered expectations young Vietnamese daughters navigated. The social control exerted over them by their immigrant parents and the community resulted in slightly higher academic achievements compared to men. Also see Kibria 1993.

32. Espin 1999; Espiritu 2001.

33. López 2002, 124.

34. González-López 2005.

35. Anzaldúa 1997, 260.

36. Telles and Ortiz 2008, 205–6.

37. Vasquez 2011.

38. See Flores 2017 for a discussion of Latinas in the teaching profession and how it has become the top occupation for Latinas with four-year college degrees. Nursing was the second-highest occupation.

39. Cabrera, Flores, and Reich, 2024.

40. González-López 2004, 1127.

CHAPTER 3

1. The definition of "first-generation college" student is murky. Some institutions define first-generation college student as anyone whose parents did not receive a bachelor's degree or equivalent in the United States. Others have more expansive definitions: students still count as first generation even when parents have a degree in another country. I define it as any student whose parents never attended college at all.

2. Becker et al. 1976; Murti 2012; Jenkins 2021; Schut 2023.

3. While requirements may vary these generally include general chemistry I and II, organic chemistry I and II with lab work, physics I and II, cell biology, molecular biology, biochemistry, human anatomy, genetics, introduction to human physiology, and one semester of calculus or a year of statistics,

4. First-generation college students often think that the only way to enter medicine is by taking courses that lead to a Bachelor of Science (BS) degree outright (K. García 2020). Most Latina/o physicians in this book thought so too as they forged their paths. However, it *is* also possible to become a doctor by obtaining bachelor's degrees in non-science related fields.

5. Flores 2011b; Taningco 2008; Cantu 2008.

6. Flores, Bañuelos and Harris, 2023; K. García 2020.

7. Talamantes et al., 2016; Albanese et al. 2003; Tiako e. al. 2021.

8. MCAT test-takers outside of the US pay an additional registration fee.

9. The current MCAT consists of four distinct sections that are individually scored: Chemical and Physical Foundations of Biological Systems, Critical Analysis and Reasoning Skills (often called CARS), Biological and Biochemical Foundations of Living Systems, and Psychological, Social and Biological Foundations of Behavior. Each section is allotted either 90 or 95 minutes and includes between 50 and 60 questions. The scoring system has changed over time.

10. Bound et al., 2021.

11. Jenkins 2021.

12. Schut 2022.

13. Powell and Kowarski 2020.

14. Vallejo 2012.

15. Secondary applications ask questions about goals, experiences, and views on several topics, including decisions for pursuing medical school. Secondary application fees range in price. They may be waived if applicants qualify for the AAMC's Fee Assistance Program.

16. Albanese et al. 2003.

17. Burton et al. 2020.

18. Tiako et al. 2021.

19. Youngclaus and Fresne 2020.

20. Puerto Rican medical schools have lower tuition costs than mainland medical schools.

21. Youngclaus and Fresne 2020.

22. Jolly 2005; Youngclaus and Fresne 2020.

23. In 2019 the self-reported median parental income of Asian students was $120,000; this number was $150,000 for Whites and $80,000 for Blacks (Youngclaus and Fresne 2020).

24. Youngclaus and Fresne 2020.

25. Gándara 1995.

26. Wingfield 2020; Murti 2012.

27. Estrada 2019; Kwon 2015; García and Flores, 2024.

28. Nicaragua became a designated country for Temporary Protected Status in 1999.

29. For more on the implications of DACA for undocumented students pursuing medical education see the Pre-Health Dreamers network (https://www.phdreamers.org). This organization currently reports over two hundred pre-health undocumented students in twenty-seven US states.

30. Abrego 2006.

31. Enriquez 2015.

32. Flores 2011b.

33. Vallejo 2012.

34. Hall and Sandler 1982; Eddy, Brownell, and Wenderoth 2014; Lee and McCabe 2021; Johnson 2012.

35. Talamantes et al., 2016.

36. Ana had three children, ages fourteen, twelve, and six.

37. A resident is a physician who has completed medical school.

38. Jacob's contact information was relayed to me from someone who knew of my project after they confirmed that it could be shared.

39. El Palacio de Justicia was in Bogota, Colombia, in Bolivar Square. It was destroyed on November 6, 1985, by M-19 guerilla warfare. Lawyers, judges, and Supreme Court justices were taken hostage during the siege.

40. To become a medical interpreter, a candidate must demonstrate fluency in at least two languages and complete formal classroom training and examinations that include medical terminology, health-care systems, sensitivity, roles/limitations, colloquialisms, and medical visits in diverse settings. Interpreters may be trained or certified. Trained medical interpreters participate in a formal education program and pass a written test to earn a certificate. They are able to work in most health-care settings. Certified interpreters go one step further and take an additional written and oral examination by the National Board of Certified Medical Interpreters (NBCMI) or the Certification Commission for Healthcare Interpreters (CCHI).

41. Five physicians had parents who were doctors who trained and worked in their countries of origin. Mario, born in the United States, was the son and grandson of men who worked as medics for bullfighters in Mexico. Gabriel was born in Chula Vista, CA, but he completed all his schooling and medical training in Universidad Autónoma de Baja California. Gabriel's father had a degree in medicine from Latin America, but he went into business instead of practicing. Mateo's father was an IMG urologist trained in Perú. Jazmín's mother was a physician in Colombia and Isabel's father was a doctor in Brazil.

42. Becker and colleagues (1976) interviewed and observed sixty-two medical students.

43. Both USMGs and IMGs are required to pass this examination before being permitted to practice medicine unsupervised. The fee for USMLE Step 1 and Step 2 Clinical Knowledge (CK) is $940 for each exam registration. The fee for Step 2 Clinical Skills (CS) is $1,580 for each exam registration.

44. Rebecca Schut (2023) defines nativist credentialism as the process whereby IMG physicians' credentials are devalued in the profession and reproduce inequality in the health spheres.

45. Irigoyen and Zambrana 1979; Feliciano 2005.

46. Dr. Maria Amarillas, a Peruvian IMG, successfully made it into the American medical system when she was offered a postdoctoral fellowship

focused on curing infectious diseases that came with a J-1 visa. She "jumped" at the opportunity. However, her "immigrant perspective" shed light on other educated South American immigrants in her circle who were doctors in Latin America and could not practice in the US. They "decided not to try or failed the exams." Maria eventually transitioned to an H-1 visa, but several of her highly educated woman peers instead became stay-at-home mothers or worked as volunteers in clinics. See the work of Daniel Dohan (2003) and Medina and Posso (2009) for an analysis of highly educated Latinos who are downwardly mobile in America.

47. Farooq 2020.

48. Rosas 2014.

49. Jenkins 2020.

50. Schut 2022.

51. Jazmín presents an interesting case of a physician who began working for marginalized communities and then expanded to work with affluent patients in Beverly Hills. In chapter 4, I examine how doctors decide to work for affluent or minority communities. For more on the Colombian diaspora see Medina et al. 2009; Guarnizo et al. 1999; Meyer et al. 1997.

52. Isabel, too, started medical school in Brazil right after high school, noting the requirements that different countries have to obtain medical degrees. "I went to medical school when I was 18 because you don't have college. You go from high school to medical school directly," she explained.

53. While Brazil is in Latin America, the country was colonized by Portugal, not Spain. However, Isabel spoke Spanish, self-identified as Latina, and was eligible to participate in the study.

54. Becker et al. 1976, 60.

55. Jenkins 2021.


CHAPTER 4

1. Portes and Fernandez-Kelly (2008) report the importance of a "really significant other," teacher, counselor, or friend of the family, as a critical factor in promoting achievement among disadvantaged children in K-12 education.

2. Stanton-Salazar 2011; Bañuelos and Flores 2021; Bashi 2007.

3. Bashi 2007.

4. Alexis Alemán and Irvin García are two Mexican heritage medical students who began the social media page *Foos in Medicine*. They chronicle their journey for other aspiring men of color who are first generation college students and feel that they do not fit the traditional "scholar" look.

5. In *Survival of the Knitted* (2007), Bashi notes that veteran migrants (hubs) act as migration experts and send for newcomers (spokes).

6. Maricela Bañuelos and I (2021) examined the forms of support that Latine doctoral students receive from various professors and how they interpreted that support as they navigated their higher educational pursuits. We found that professors of various racial/ethnic backgrounds provide institutional support. However, Latine doctoral students narrated that their social capital was bolstered by Latine professors' networks and instrumental support by way of their possession of relevant experiential knowledge and a critical consciousness.

7. Stanton-Sálazar 2011.

8. Tiako, Ray and South 2022; Flores 2017.

9. Tiako, Ray and South 2022.

10. Ivan explained that unlike most medical students, he only applied to one school.

11. Armando had married a US citizen, an Asian-American physician, but the Defense of Marriage Act (DOMA) presented unique obstacles for the same-sex couple due to his foreign-born status. His experience of difficulties navigating visa requirements is typical of international medical graduates (Jenkins 2021).

12. For more on foreign-trained STEM professionals working in technical industries in the United States see Banerjee and Rincón 2019.

13. Jenkins 2021.

14. Bourdieu 1984; Stanton-Salazar 2011; Rosales 2020.

15. Bañuelos and Flores 2021; Cantú 2006.

16. Hurtado 2006. Chicana feminist scholars use testimonios as a qualitative methodological tool and mode of inquiry.

17. Samuel's parents attended college in Perú but did not finish. His father was studying to be an engineer and his mother was studying to be an accountant. His grandmother worked in obstetrics and physical therapy in Perú.

18. Rendon 2019.

19. Bashi 2007.

20. Stanton-Salazar and Dornbusch 1995; Zhou and Kim 2006.

21. Rendón et al. 2019.

22. This is a pseudonym.

23. Premedical students are not obligated to shadow a physician in order to qualify for medical school. However, first-generation college students who did not have high status connections to medicine indicated this was crucial to gaining important clinical experience. The number of shadowing hours can vary.

24. Lee and Hatteberg 2015.

25. Smith 2005.

26. García and Flores, forthcoming. In chapter 5, I explain how much of this translating and interpretation work becomes gendered; Latina doctors are much more overburdened with this work than their male counterparts.

27. Portes and Fernández Kelly 2008.

28. Other programs, such as Pre-Health Dreamers, catered specifically to undocumented students pursuing medicine and provided a wealth of information on ways to navigate different bureaucracies.

29. Another post-graduate program is The Society for Advancement of Chicanos/Hispanics and Native Americans in Science (SACNAS).

30. García and Flores, forthcoming.

31. García 2022.

32. In exchange for scholarship support, recipients must serve a minimum of two years at a NHSC-approved site in a Health Professional Shortage Area.

33. Talamantes et al., 2016.

34. N. López 2002.

35. Ophthalmologists perform medical and surgical procedures for eye conditions while optometrists examine and treat a patient's eyes.

36. See Teherani et al. (2018) for more on differences in clinical performance evaluations and how this determines who gets awards and honors which influence residency selection and career choices. The authors call this amplification cascade.

37. Failing one rotation does not mean that someone is automatically removed from a program, but it could. Medical school personnel usually decide the course of action they will take.

38. Cassell 1998, 100.

39. AAMC 2022.

40. Vallejo 2012.

41. Cantú 2006.

42. Gina García (2019) notes that several institutions of higher education have obtained HSI status for enrolling Latinx students but do not necessarily serve their unique educational needs.

## CHAPTER 5

1. Acker 1990; 2006.

2. Ong 2005.

3. Goffman 1956, 476.

4. For instance, as white women doctors entered medicine, they were initially gender-typed into less lucrative specialties and snubbed by some white men doctors and nurses (see Cassell 1997).

5. A. Padilla 1994; Wingfield 2019.

6. Misra et al. 2024.

7. Murti 2012.

8. Vega et. al. 2010; Mendoza, Masuda, and Swartout 2015.

9. Alfrey and Twine 2017.

10. Alegria 2019.

11. In a previous project on Latina teachers who work as numerical tokens among a majority of white teachers (Flores 2017), I used the concept *racialized tokens* to highlight the inequities they experienced on the job.

12. Registered nurses who reported being Asian accounted for 7.2 percent of the workforce, representing the largest non-white racial group. African Americans were 6.7 percent (Smiley et. al., 2021). For a more detailed analysis of the barriers that Latinas/os describe in their trajectories into nursing, see Vogt and Taningco 2008. Lack of time to study due to family obligations, financial support, and lack of academic preparation were reported as key obstacles.

13. Molina, Landry, Chary, and Burnett-Bowie (2020), four women of color physicians, note that nurses accept similar orders from male residents without question. They surmise it is due to not trusting the female resident's clinical acumen. It is important to note that nurses often feel disrespected by physicians, and studies have called for the need to improve nurse-physician collaboration.

14. Cassell 1997, 50.

15. Such is the case in Kwon and Adams's (2018) assessment of Asian-Canadian women medical professionals in training who were advised by white women colleagues to remain "humble" to avoid negative interactions with nurses. It can also be seen in a study of Latinas pursuing medicine who experience sexually derogatory comments linked to ethnicity (Grijalva and Coombs 1997).

16. Reskin and Roos (1990) introduced the queuing perspective to describe white women's entrance into male-dominated workplaces. Their model describes the uneven distribution of groups across occupations as the result of a dual queuing process: labor queues that order groups of workers in terms of their attractiveness to employers, and job queues in which workers rank themselves.

17. Ridgeway 2014.

18. Zelek and Phillips 2003.

19. Female chaperones are required to be in the room when physicians are performing certain exams to ensure the patient's comfort and to support and protect doctors.

20. Solórzano and Yosso 2000.

21. García-López and Segura 2008.

22. Valian 1999, 15.

23. García-López and Segura 2008.

24. For more on the impact of age on professional Latinas see the work of Shannon Portillo (2010).

25. Ridgeway 2014.

26. Pierce 1995a.

27. Cassell 1998.

28. Saraswati 2023.

29. A. Padilla 1994.


CHAPTER 6

1. Soraida's hometown was in Naguabo. Her mother obtained a scholarship to complete a PhD in Chemistry at NYU but was unable to attend. Her father passed away during this time and as the eldest daughter she had to return to

the island to help her mother raise her siblings. Still, Soraida's mother became the superintendent of a school district. When her father lived, he enrolled in the military and later worked as a policeman in Puerto Rico.

2. For more on Afro-Latines in medicine read up on Dr. José Celso Barbosa (1857–1921), who was the first Black Puerto Rican physician to earn a medical degree in the United States. As I worked on this book, I also became aware that a Puerto Rican, Afro-Latina mother-daughter duo was featured on season 17 of the popular medical show *Grey's Anatomy,* although their roles were minor.

3. Puerto Ricans are part of the island *and* the mainland as a common-wealth of the United States. The Jones Act of 1917 granted US citizenship to all Puerto Ricans. Unlike other Latino subgroups that faced more draconian exclusionary immigration policies, she experienced regular movement between the two territories. Ariana Valle (2019) argues that Puerto Ricans experience what she calls a colonial/racialized citizenship in America.

4. Bonilla-Silva 2004.

5. She mentioned Ahmaud Marquez Arbery (May 8, 1994–February 23, 2020) and George Perry Floyd Jr. (October 14, 1973–May 25, 2020).

6. Monk 2021.

7. Dixon and Telles 2017.

8. Roth 2016.

9. I use the term white-presenting because even though these Latino professionals might have noted "white" on the race question on United States census forms, none of them identified as white socially.

10. Picca and Feagin 2007.

11. Similarly, Ayu Saraswati (2013) notes that ethnicity complicates how colorism is understood among Asian Americans.

12. Perhaps because I focused my project on physicians in California, I had trouble recruiting Afro-Latine doctors. I suspect that if I had expanded my study to include physicians on the East Coast or Florida, I may have come across more Black Cuban or Dominican physicians. Migration patterns, however, show that it was the Golden Cuban Exiles (1959–1962) that had a large share of highly educated and lighter skinned Cubans, some of whom were doctors and settled in Florida.

13. I make a distinction between Latin American doctors who said they were white, and US-born or raised Latinas/os who indicated they were

phenotypically fairer-skinned and reported being able to pass. They recognized the benefits of being mistaken for white but did not see themselves as racially white due to racialization process of Latines in the US.

14. Jorge Duany (1998) discusses these categorizations in Puerto Rico and the Dominican Republic, and Sylvia Zamora (2022) focuses on Mexico.

15. Ostfeld and Yadon (2021) evaluated the extent to which respondents saw themselves as darker or lighter, providing insight into the effects of perceptions on lived experiences. They found that Latino-Americans who rated themselves as lighter and/or overestimated their lightness held fewer liberal positions on contemporary racialized issues. Conversely, those who rated themselves as darker and/or overestimated their skin darkness took a more liberal position on racialized political issues. For more also see Hannon and DeFina 2016.

16. Hargrove and Gonzalez 2022.

17. Noe-Bustamante et al., 2021.

18. Podiatrists are doctors but they do not attend traditional medical schools. DPM (doctor of podiatric medicine) appears after their name instead of MD.

19. For more on how the children of immigrants serve as language brokers for the immigrant parents see Delgado (2020) and Kwon (2015).

20. Roth 2016.

21. Rincón et al. 2020.

22. Rincón 2015; Rincón et al. 2020.

23. Rincón et al. 2020.

24. Rincón (2017) argues that regardless of educational background, immigration law places all migrants with temporary legal statuses in a system of stratification that economically and socially marginalizes them. High-skilled immigrants of color face precarity, legal violence, stereotyping, exploitation, and long, anxious waits (Banerjee and Rincón 2019). It is worth noting that Rincón's interviewees linked this anxiety and fear to the uncertainty of their temporary legal status and not to experiences of criminalization based on racial assumptions, as is the case with Central American and other Latine migrants (Golash Boza and Hondagneu-Sotelo 2013; Ménjivar and Abrego 2012).

25. N. López 2002; Gutiérrez 2008.

26. Picca and Feagin 2007.

27. Microaggressions are verbal or behavioral snubs or slights that may be intentional or unintentional (Sue 2010).

28. See Lugo-Lugo (2008) for a more thorough discussion of the complicated nature of using mestizaje to characterize multiple Latine subgroups.

29. Acuña 1996.

30. Wingfield 2019.

31. Murti 2014.

32. Ochoa 2013.

33. Asian Americans are also internally stratified. The model minority myth also hurts Asians who may be of lower socioeconomic status and need more resources to succeed.

34. Hsin and Xie 2014.

35. Lee and Zhou 2015.

36. Kochnar and Cilluffo 2018.

37. Mukkamala and Suyemoto 2018.

38. According to Lu et al. (2020), South Asians were more likely to experience ethnic hostility and racial profiling in the aftermath of 9/11. Meanwhile anti-Asian hate crimes grew considerably during the COVID-19 pandemic in 2020.

39. For more on the bamboo ceiling see Hyun 2005; Lu et al. 2020.

40. For more on Asians in the health industry, such as Filipina nurses, see the work of Catherine Ceniza Choy (2003) and Yen Le Espiritu (2003).

41. See Pérez 2022.

42. Wingfield 2012.

43. According to Patricia Hill Collins (2000), controlling images are more than just racial stereotypes because they have the power to influence rules and policymaking. One controlling image that was applied to Latinas was that of hyperfertility, which at times has caused the forced sterilization of Mexican immigrant women and Puerto Rican women. For more on this topic see Espino and Tajima-Peña 2016.

44. Vasquez-Tokos and Norton-Smith 2016; Collins 2020.

45. Vallejo 2012.

46. Noe-Bustamante et al. 2021.

47. Hargrove and Gonzalez 2022.

48. Bonilla-Silva 2004.

49. Indeed, Dr. Maria Amarillas, a Peruvian IMG, noted how her conceptions of color changed while attending an expensive private medical school in her home country, where she was exposed to more white male medical

students. These interactions prepared her for what she would encounter in American medical workplaces. She said, "In Perú color isn't such a common thing [for racial classification]. I never really had that question growing up. I was just Peruvian. But, ever since I've been living here [in the U.S.] I have to say 'I am Latino or mixed race.' At least in Perú the majority of us are some shade of brown and so we're all mestizo. I am brown but not super dark. Maybe I am darker than the average white, male student in a private medical school. Anytime I would enter a room [in medical school in Perú], I was always their nurse, the housekeeper, never the doctor. Even in Perú, if there were guys no matter the color, especially if they were blue-eyed and blond, they were always the doctors even though they were medical students."

50. Indeed, Cuban anthropologist Jorge Duany (1998) argues that migrants bring their cultural conceptions of their identity, which often do not match those of the host society. This is especially the case for Caribbean migrants. An example would be Dominicans in the Dominican Republic, who perceive Haitians as the other. Also see Waters 2001.

51. Williams 1992.


CHAPTER 7

1. I have changed the name of the practice to protect Perla's identity and that of her patients.

2. Up to 40 percent of white medical trainees believe that Black people have "thicker skin" and are less sensitive to pain than white people, which can lead to less-than-optimal treatment of pain in Black patients (Hoffman et al. 2016). Murtha and Bekiesz (2022) discuss how a critical race theory perspective can help trainees understand race as a social construction in health.

3. In chapter 5 I explain Perla's reasons for opening her own practice in detail, but the ability to hire and train the office staff who would help her provide her patients with care was primary.

4. Several Latina MDs who were married indicated that their husbands had lower levels of education and made less money than they did. In some cases, they had made the decision as a family unit that their husband would be a stay-at-home parent. This led to unique family dynamics, especially when the women were the children of immigrants. For an analysis of how professional

or immigration status alters the gendered division of household labor see Pesquera 1993 and Hondagneu-Sotelo 1992.

5. Perla would see ten to fifteen patients in thirty-minute blocks every day, a time she stuck to or else it would cut into the next person's appointment and cause her to fall behind. At times she would shorten or forego lunch to try and squeeze in an extra patient.

6. Metzl and Hansen 2014.

7. Holmes 2013.

8. Zewude and Sharma 2020; Solorzano and Yosso 2002.

9. Metzl and Hansen 2014.

10. Olszweski 2022, 213.

11. Latina/o doctors asked seventeen patients if I could be in the room. One woman declined.

12. Clinicians who worked in migrant clinics that kept paper records in Holmes's (2013) study described the medical records of Latino/a immigrants as "patchy." They seemed unaware that seasonal migrant work schedules meant that many workers receive care in scattered settings.

13. While some doctors might interpret *me duele mi pecho* [my chest hurts] as indicative of a heart attack, Cipriano was signaling the severity of his cough and its effects on his diaphragm.

14. *Ire* is Mexican slang for *"mire,"* look!.

15. López et al., 2022; Funk and López 2022.

16. Raudenbush 2021.

17. The rest of the standards can be accessed at https://minorityhealth.hhs.gov/assets/pdf/checked/finalreport.pdf.

18. Family members often accompany one another to a provider's office, especially when treatment is invasive or out of the ordinary. This practice disproportionately affects racialized people and families. Several studies have pointed this out. See Zewude and Sharma 2020; Corona et al. 2012; Kwon 2015; García and Flores, forthcoming.

19. In Latin America, it is customary to first jot down the day and then the month, often causing confusion in the US, as a Latina doctor pointed out when she noticed an incorrect birth date for a child.

20. Laundry Workers Center 2018. Some workers reported buying their own safety equipment.

21. Funk and López 2022.

22. Holmes 2012.

23. Torres et al., 2022.

24. Tsai and Crawford-Roberts 2017.

25. Jenks 2011.

26. Holmes 2013.

27. For more on cultural competency and health policy see Kaplan and Zavaleta's (2017) commentary piece in the Harvard Kennedy School's *Journal of Hispanic Policy*.

28. Fadiman 2012.

29. Holmes 2012.

30. Zewude and Sharma 2021.

31. Becker et al. 1961, 322.

32. Spanish conversational language codes among working-class Latino immigrant parents and Latina teachers—most of whom were children of immigrants or, if they were not born in the United States, came here as children—contained a wide range of such switches.

33. The medical Spanish coursework offered by the Instituto Cultural Oaxaca covers three different modules.

34. Maria looked up *culebrilla*. Hayes-Bautista and Chiprut's (2008) book has an excellent glossary of Latine cultural understandings that practitioners may find useful.

35. Elderkin-Thomson, Silver, and Waitzin 2001; Rodarte et al. 2024.

36. Rafferty, Tsikoudas, and Davis 2007.

37. Spanish linguist Dalia Magaña (2021) has an excellent book that discusses the importance of different forms of communication with Latine patients.

38. Hunt 2005.

39. Gálvez 2018.

40. García and Flores, forthcoming.

41. Gálvez 2018.

42. Cunningham et al. 2021.

43. Loizate 2009.

44. The first time that I had observed Dr. Lisa Macias she was wearing her white coat. But this time she wasn't; instead she was wearing a black Mexican

peasant blouse with colorful flowers, blue pants, loafers, and her hair was down. Her many tattoos were exposed.

45. Julliard and colleagues (2008) discuss that Latina patients might not disclose important information to their providers, especially around issues of sexuality or genital examination. We see evidence of this when the Latina immigrant patient verifies if everyone in the room is a woman, and then affirms that Lisa and Pushpa can examine her because they are all women.

46. The birthdate on the child's file was wrong. Lisa made the changes to the file. See Estrada et al. (2019) who discuss how immigration is a social determinant of health that shapes doctor-patient interactions.

47. Flores 2020a.

48. On January 1, 2024, undocumented immigrants between the ages of twenty-six and forty-nine became eligible for Medi-Cal in the state of California. Unfortunately, people like Fidel did not qualify for the state's Medicaid program ten years ago. He could not access a specialist.

49. Holmes 2013.

50. The California Medical Assistance Program is the California implementation of the federal Medicaid program serving low-income individuals, including families, seniors, persons with disabilities, children in foster care, pregnant women, and childless adults with incomes below 138 percent of the federal poverty level.

51. Holmes 2013.

52. Fernander 2022.


## CHAPTER 8

1. Dill and Salsberg 2008.

2. We should go beyond the gender binary and extend this to LGBTQ+ people, too.

3. Browne, Tatum, and Gonzalez 2021.

4. Dr. Valentina Peralta, in family medicine, was the other Cuban American in the sample. Her parents also settled in Los Angeles upon US arrival, but they were highly educated immigrants. Valentina narrated that her parents "left Cuba for political freedom."

5. The US-born child of poor Cuban immigrants who made their home in East Los Angeles, a departure from prior waves that settled in Florida, Enrique

thoroughly enjoyed his undergraduate and medical school experience at the University of Miami and University of Florida, respectively.

6. Guo and Nambudiri 2021.

7. AAMC 2022.

8. World Health Organization 2023.

9. Pérez and Reis da Silva 2019; Burke 2013. Several other scholars and medical professionals have also examined what the feminization of their physician workforce means for health providers and patients. See Levinson and Lurie (2004) for an examination of Canadian doctors and Bedoya-Vaca, Derose, and Rombero-Sandoval (2016) for an exploration of these dynamics in Ecuador.

10. Medical anthropologists have pointed out the shifts of food access and shortage over time on the island. For a detailed analysis see Garth 2020.

11. I do not include Arianny (a pseudonym) in my overall sample count, as she did not meet the eligibility criteria. I do include an abridged version of our discussion because it provides an interesting contrast to what US Latina/o doctors face and bolsters the overall analysis of the book. In my immigration forms I marked "research" as the reason for the trip.

12. According to Emma, I would be considered a *trigueña* or *india* in the racial classification system on the island.

13. Augustin 2020.

14. Burke 2013.

# References

Abrego, Leisy. 2006. ""I Can't go to College Because I Don't Have Papers': Incorporation Patterns of Latino Undocumented Youth." *Latino Studies* 4: 212–31.

———. 2014. *Sacrificing Families: Navigating Laws, Labor, and Love across Borders*. Stanford: Stanford University Press.

Acker, Joan. 1990. "Hierarchies, Jobs, Bodies: A Theory of Gendered Organizations." *Gender and Society* 4: 139–58.

———. 2006. "Inequality Regimes: Gender, Class, and Race in Organizations." *Gender & Society* 20(4): 441–64.

Acuña, Rodolfo F. 1996. *Anything But Mexican: Chicanos in Contemporary Los Angeles*. London and New York: Verso Books.

Ahn, Taemin, Hector De Leon, Misael Galdámez, Ana Oaxaca, Rocio Perez, Denise Ramos-Vega, Lupe Renteria Salome, and Jie Zong. 2022. "15 Facts About Latino Well-Being in California." Los Angeles, CA: UCLA Latino Policy and Politics Institute.

Albanese, Mark A., Mikel H. Snow, Susan E. Skochelak, Kathryn N. Huggett, and Philip M. Farrell. 2003. "Assessing Personal Qualities in Medical School Admissions." *Academic Medicine* 78(3): 313–21.

Alegria, Sharla. 2019. "Escalator or Step Stool? Gendered Labor and Token Processes in Tech Work." *Gender and Society* 33(5): 722–45.

Alfrey, Lauren, and France Winddance Twine. 2017. "Gender-Fluid Geek Girls: Negotiating Inequality Regimes in the Tech Industry." *Gender and Society* 31(1): 28–50.

Anaya, Yohualli B., Paul Hsu, Laura E. Martinez, Stephanie Hernandez, and David Hayes-Bautista. 2022. "Latina Women in the U.S. Physician Workforce: Opportunities in the Pursuit of Health Equity." *Association of American Medical Colleges* 97(3): 398–405.

Anaya, Yohualli B., Paul Hsu, Seira Santizo Greenwood, and David Hayes-Bautista. 2023. "Improvement Needed in Latina Physician Representation: Implications for Medical Education, Training, and Policy." UCLA Latino Policy & Politics Institute.

Anzaldúa, Gloria. 1997. "Movimientos de Rebeldia y las Culturas que Traicionan." In *Latinos and Education,* edited by Antonia Darder and Rodolfo D. Torres, 259–268. New York: Routledge.

Association of American Medical Colleges. 2014. "Diversity in the Physician Workforce." Accessed July 24, 2018. https://aamcdiversityfactsandfigures .org/section-iii-geographic-distribution-of-physician-workforce.

———. 2018. "Diversity in Medicine: Facts and Figures." Accessed February 26, 2020. https://www.aamc.org/data-reports/workforce/interactive-data /figure-18-percentage-all-active-physicians-race/ethnicity-2018.

———. 2022a. "Diversity Facts & Figures." https://www.aamc. org/data-reports/workforce/report/diversity-facts-figures.

———. 2022b. "State Physician Workforce Data Report." https://store.aamc .org/2021-state-physician-workforce-data-report.html.

———. 2023. "Table B-6.1: Total Graduates by U.S. MD-Granting Medical School and Race/Ethnicity (Alone), 2022–2023." https://www.aamc.org /media/6126/download.

Augustin, Ed. 2020. "Cuba Has Sent 2,000 Doctors and Nurses Overseas to Fight Covid-19." *The Nation*. Accessed on October 16, 2023. https://www .thenation.com/article/world/cuba-doctors-covid-19.

Becker, Howard S., Blanche Geer, Everett C. Hughes, and Anselm L. Strauss. 1976. *Boys in White: Student Culture in Medical School*. London: Routledge.

Banerjee, Pallavi, and Lina Rincón. 2019. "Trouble in Tech Paradise." *Contexts* 18(2): 24–29.

Bañuelos, Maricela, and Glenda M. Flores. 2021. ""I Could See Myself": Professors' Influence in First-Generation Latinx College Students' Pathways into Doctoral Programs." *Race, Ethnicity & Education* 27(5): 599–619.

Bashi, Vilna. 2007. *Survival of the Knitted: Immigrant Social Networks in a Stratified World*. Palo Alto, CA: Stanford University Press.

Basu, Sanjay, et al. 2019. "Association of Primary Care Physician Supply with Population Mortality in the United States, 2005–2015." *JAMA Intern Med* 179(4): 506–14.

Beagan, Brenda. 2001. "Micro Inequities and Everyday Inequalities: Race, Gender, Sexuality and Class in Medical School." *The Canadian Journal of Sociology* 22(4): 583–610.

Bettie, Julie. 2003. *Women without Class: Girls, Race, and Identity*. Berkeley: University of California Press.

Bedoya-Vaca, Rita, Kathryn P. Derose and Natalia Romero-Sandoval. 2016. "Gender and Physician Specialization and Practice Settings in Ecuador: A Qualitative Study." *BMC Health Services Research* 16: 662, https://doi.org/10.1186/s12913-016-1917-1.

Bhatt, Wasudha. 2013. "The Little Brown Woman: Gender Discrimination in American Medicine." *Gender and Society* 27(5): 659–80.

Bonilla-Silva, Eduardo. 2004. "From Bi-racial to Tri-racial: Towards a New System of Racial Stratification in the USA." *Ethnic and Racial Studies* 27(6): 931–50.

Bourdieu, Pierre. 1984. *The Forms of Capital. Excerpt from Distinction: A Social Critique of the Judgment of Taste*. Translated by Richard Nice. Cambridge, MA: Harvard University Press.

Brewer, Alexandra, Melissa Osborne, Anna S. Mueller, Daniel M. O'Connor, Arjun Dayal, and Vineet M. Arora. 2020. "Who Gets the Benefit of the Doubt? Performance Evaluations, Medical Errors, and the Production of Gender Inequality in Emergency Medical Education." *American Sociological Review* 85(2): 247–70.

Browne, Irene, Katherine Tatum, and Belisa Gonzalez. 2021. "Presumed Mexican Until Proven Otherwise: Identity Work and Intersectional Typicality

Among Middle-Class Dominican and Mexican Immigrants." *Social Problems* 68(5): 80–99.

Bound, John, Breno Braga, Gaurav Khanna, and Sarah Turner. 2021. "The Globalization of Postsecondary Education: The Role of International Students in the US Higher Education System." *Journal of Economic Perspectives* 35(1): 163–84.

Burke, Nancy. 2013. *Health Travels: Cuban Health(care) On and Off the Island.* Berkeley: University of California Medical Humanities Press.

Burton, Brittany N., Angele S. Labastide, Bannet N. Muhoozi, Christian G. Lopez-Ramos, Alpha T. Anders, Katherine Garcia, Rodney A. Gabriel, and Lindia Willies-Jacobo. 2020. "Socioeconomic Status and Mock Interview Performance among Prospective Medical School Applicants." *Journal of Health Care for the Poor and Underserved* 31(1): 105–14.

Cabrera, Jennifer, Glenda M. Flores, and Stephanie Reich. 2024. "Gendered Cultural Tightropes: Bicultural Latinas Navigating and Negotiating *Familismo* in American Doctoral Programs." *Gender and Education* 36(6): 564–80.

Cantu, Norma. 2008. *Paths to Discovery: Autobiographies from Chicanas with Careers in Science, Mathematics, and Engineering.* UCLA Chicano Studies Research Center Press.

Cantu, Norma, ed. 2006. *Flor y Ciencia: Chicanas in Science, Mathematics and Engineering.* Washington, DC: The Adelante Project, AAAS.

Cassell, Joan. 1997. "Doing Gender, Doing Surgery: Women Surgeons in a Man's Profession." *Human Organization* 56(1): 47–52.

———. 1998. *The Woman in the Surgeon's Body.* Cambridge: Harvard University Press.

Chávez, Maria. 2011. *Everyday Injustice: Latino Professionals and Racism.* Lanham, MD: Rowman & Littlefield.

———. 2019. *Latina Professionals in America: Testimonios of Policy, Perseverance, and Success.* London: Routledge.

Choy, Catherine Ceniza. 2003. *Empire of Care: Nursing and Migration in Filipino American History.* Durham, NC: Duke University Press.

Collins, Patricia Hill. 2019. *Intersectionality as Critical Social Theory.* Durham: Duke University Press.

———. 2000. *Black Feminist Thought: Knowledge, Consciousness, and the Politics of Empowerment.* New York: Routledge.

Corona, Rosalie, Lillian F. Stevens, Raquel W. Halfond, Carla M. Shaffer, Kathryn Reid-Quiñones, and Tanya Gonzalez. 2012. "A Qualitative Analysis of What Latino Parents and Adolescents Think and Feel About Language Brokering." *Journal of Child and Family Studies* 21(5): 788–98.

Crenshaw, Kimberlé. 1991. "Mapping the Margins: Intersectionality, Identity Politics, and Violence Against Women of Color." *Stanford Law Review* 43(6): 1241–99.

Cunningham, Amy, Denine Crittendon, Casey Konys, Geoffrey Mills, Allison Casola, Samantha Kelly, and Christine Arenson. 2021. "Critical Race Theory as a Lens for Examining Primary Care Provider Responses to Persistently-Elevated HbA1c." *Journal of the National Medical Association* 113(3): 297–300.

Dasgupta, Shamita Das, and Sayantani DasGupta. 1996. "Public Face, Private Space: Asian Indian Women and Sexuality." In *"Bad Girls"/"Good Girls": Women, Sex, and Power in the Nineties,* edited by Nan Bauer-Maglin and Donna Perry, 226–46. New Brunswick: Rutgers University Press.

Delgado, Vanessa. 2020. "Decoding the Hidden Curriculum: Latina/o First-Generation College Students' Influence on Young Siblings' Educational Trajectory." *Journal of Latinos and Education* 22(2): 624–41.

Dill, Michael J., and Edward S. Salsberg. 2008. "The Complexities of Physician Supply and Demand: Projections through 2025." *Association of American Medical Colleges.* Washington, DC: AAMC.

Dixon, Angela R., and Edward E. Telles. 2017. "Skin Color and Colorism: Global Research, Concepts, and Measurement." *Annual Review of Sociology* 43: 405–24.

Dohan, Daniel. 2003. *The Price of Poverty.* Berkeley: University of California Press.

Duany, Jorge. 1998. "Reconstructing Racial Identity: Ethnicity, Color and Class among Dominicans in the United States and Puerto Rico." *Latin American Perspectives* 25(3): 147–72.

Eddy, Sarah L., Sara E. Brownell, and Mary Pat Wenderoth. 2014. "Gender Gaps in Achievement and Participation in Multiple Introductory Biology Classrooms." *CBE Life Science Education* 13(3): 478–92.

Elderkin-Thompson, Virginia, Roxane Cohen Silver, and Howard Waitzkin. 2021. "When Nurses Double as Interpreters: A Study of Spanish-Speaking Patients in a US Primary Care Setting." *Social Science and Medicine* 52(9): 1343–58.

Enloe, Cynthia. 2004. *The Curious Feminist: Searching for Women in a New Age of Empire*. Berkeley: University of California Press.

Enriquez, Laura. 2015. "Multigenerational Punishment: Shared Experiences of Undocumented Immigration Status Within Mixed-Status Families." *Journal of Marriage and Family* 77(4): 939–53.

Espin, Olivia. 1999. *Women Crossing Boundaries: A Psychology of Immigration and Transformations of Sexuality*. New York: Routledge Press.

Espino, Virginia, producer, and Renee Tajima-Peña, dir. 2016. *No Más Bebés*. Los Angeles, California: Moon Canyon Films and the Independent Television Series.

Espiritu, Yen Le. 1993. *Asian American Panethnicity: Bridging Institutions and Identities*. Philadelphia: Temple University Press.

———. 2001. "'We don't sleep around like white girls do': Family, culture and gender in Filipina American lives." *Signs* 26(2): 415–40.

———. 2003. *Home Bound: Filipino American Lives across Cultures, Communities, and Countries*. Berkeley: University of California Press.

Estrada, Allison, Lilian Milanes, Roshni Kakaiya, Aisha Van Pratt Levin, Ana Ortiz, Cecilia Vazquez, and Shaila Serpas. 2019. "Family Physicians Have a Role in Care of Undocumented Patients." American Academy of Family Physicians. https://www.aafp.org/news/opinion/20191209guested-undocumented.html.

Estrada, Emir. 2013. "Changing Household Dynamics: Children's American Generational Resources in Street Vending Markets." *Childhoods* 20(1): 51–65.

———. 2019. *Kids at Work: Latinx Families Selling Food on the Streets of Los Angeles*. New York: NYU Press.

Estrada, Emir, and Pierrette Hondagneu-Sotelo. 2013. "Living the Third Shift: Latina Adolescent Street Vendors in Los Angeles." In *Immigrant Women Workers in the Neoliberal Age*, edited by Nilda Flores-Gonzalez, Anna Romina Guevarra, and Maura Toro-Morn, 144–63. Urbana: University of Illinois Press.

Fadiman, Anne. 2012. *The Spirit Catches You and You Fall Down: A Hmong Child, Her American Doctors, and the Collision of Two Cultures*. New York: Farrar, Strauss and Giroux.

Falcón, Sylvanna. 2008. "Mestiza Double Consciousness: The Voices of Afro-Peruvian Women on Gendered Racism." *Gender & Society* 22(5): 660–80.

Farooq, Yasmin Ghazala. 2020. *Elite Migrants: South Asian Doctors in the UK*. London: Transnational Press.

Feliciano, Cynthia. 2005. *Unequal Origins: Immigrant Selection and the Education of the Second Generation*. New York: LFB Scholarly Publishing.

Fernander, Anita. 2022. "What Does Critical Race Theory Have to Do with Academic Medicine?" *Journal of the National Medical Association* 114(3): 274–77.

Fernandez-Kelly, Maria Patricia, and Anna Garcia. 1997. "Power Surrendered, Power Restored: The Politics of Work and Family Among Garment Workers in Southern California and Southern Florida." In *Challenging Fronteras*, edited by Mary Romero, Pierrette Hondagneu-Sotelo, and Vilma Ortiz, 215–28. New York: Routledge.

Flores, Glenda M. 2017. *Latina Teachers: Creating Careers and Guarding Culture*. New York: New York University Press.

———. 2019. "Pursuing *Medicina* [Medicine]: Latina Physicians and Parental Messages on Gendered Career Choices." *Sex Roles* 81: 59–73.

———. 2020a. "Latina Physicians as 'Essential' Workers." *Contexts* 19(4): 62–64.

———. 2020b. "Latina/x *Doctoras* [Doctors]: Negotiating Knowledge Production in Science." In *Introduction to Women's, Gender, and Sexuality Studies: Interdisciplinary and Intersectional Approaches*, 2nd ed., edited by L. Ayu Saraswati, Barbara L. Shaw, and Heather Rellihan, 455–59. Oxford: Oxford University Press.

———. 2011a. "Racialized Tokens: Latina Teachers Negotiating, Surviving and Thriving in a White Woman's Profession." *Qualitative Sociology* 32(4): 313–35.

———. 2011b. "Latino/as in the Hard Sciences: Increasing Latina/o Participation in Science, Technology, Engineering and Math (STEM) Fields." *Latino Studies* 9: 327–35.

Flores, Glenda M., and Maricela Bañuelos. 2021. "Gendered Deference: Perceptions of Authority and Competence Among Latina/o Physicians in Medical Institutions." *Gender & Society* 35(1): 110–35.

Flores, Glenda M., Maricela Bañuelos and Pheather R. Harris. 2023. "What Are You Doing Here?: Examining Minoritized Student Undergraduate Experiences in STEM at a Minority Serving Institution." *Journal for STEM Education Research* 7: 181–204.

Foucault, Michel. 1994 [1963]. *The Birth of the Clinic: An Archaeology of Medical Perception*. New York: Vintage Press.

Funk, Cary, and Mark Hugo López. 2022. "Hispanic Americans' Trust in and Engagement with Science." Washington, DC: Pew Research Center.

Gálvez, Alyshia. 2018. *Eating Nafta: Trade, Food Policies, and the Destruction of Mexico*. Berkeley: University of California Press.

Gándara, Patricia. 1995. *Over the Ivy Walls: The Educational Mobility of Low Income Chicanos*. Albany: SUNY Press.

García, Ana Maria, dir. 1982. *La Operación*. Latin American Film Project.

García, Gina Ann. 2019. *Becoming Hispanic-Serving Institutions: Opportunities for Colleges and Universities*. Baltimore, MD: Johns Hopkins University Press.

García, Katherine A. 2020. "A Latina pursuing her medical dream (MD)." *InterActions: UCLA Journal of Education and Information Studies* 16(2): https://doi.org/10.5070/D4162046052.

——. 2022. "Impact of COVID-19 Pandemic on the Future Generation of Latinx Physicians." *Journal of Latinos and Education* 21(3): 335–45.

García, Katherine, and Glenda M. Flores. forthcoming. "Mamá en inglés se dice 'pre-Med'": Bilingual Mexican-Origin First-Generation College Undergraduates Aspiring for Medical Careers." *Race, Ethnicity & Education*. DOI: 10.1080/13613324.2024.2349879.

García, Lorena. 2012. *Respect Yourself, Protect Yourself: Latina Girls and Sexual Identity*. New York: New York University Press.

García-López, Gladys, and Denise Segura. 2008. "'They Are Testing You All the Time': Negotiating Dual Femininities among Chicana Attorneys." *Feminist Studies* 34: 229–58.

Garth, Hannah. 2020. *Food in Cuba: The Pursuit of a Decent Meal*. Stanford, CA: Stanford University Press.

Geiger, Gabriella, Lauren Kiel, Miki Horiguchi, Celia Martinez-Aceves, Kelly Meza, Briana Christophers, Priscilla Orellana, Maria Mora Pinzon, Sam J. Lubner, and Narjust Flores. 2024. "Latinas in Medicine: Evaluating and Understanding the Experience of Latinas in Medical Education: A Cross Sectional Survey. *BMC Medical Education* 24(4): 1–7.

Goffman, Erving. 1956. "The Nature of Deference and Demeanor." *American Anthropologist* 58(3): 473–502.

Golash-Boza, Tanya, and Pierrette Hondagneu-Sotelo. 2013. "Latino Immigrant Men and the Deportation Crisis: A Gendered Racial Removal Program." *Latino Studies* 11(3): 271–92.

Golden, Daniel. 2005. *The Price of Admission: How America's Ruling Class Buys Its Way into Elite Colleges—and Who Gets Left Outside the Gates.* New York: Crown Publishing Group.

González-López, Gloria. 2004. "Fathering Latina Sexualities: Mexican Men and the Virginity of Their Daughters." *Journal of Marriage and Family* 66(5): 1118–30.

———. 2005. *Erotic Journeys: Mexican Immigrants and Their Sex Lives.* Berkeley: University of California Press.

Goshua, Anna. 2019. "The Weight of the White Coat." *Journal of the American Medical Association* 321(1): 35–36.

Grijalva, Cindy A., and Robert Holman Coombs. 1997. "Latinas in Medicine: Stressors, Survival Skills, and Strengths." *Aztlán: A Journal of Chicano Studies* 22(2): 67–88.

Guarnizo, Luis Eduardo, Arturo Ignacio Sánchez, and Elizabeth M. Roach. 1999. "Mistrust, Fragmented Solidarity, and Transnational Migration: Colombians in New York City and Los Angeles." *Ethnic and Racial Studies* 22(2): 367–96.

Guo, Lisa N., and Vinod E. Nambudiri. 2021. "International Medical Graduates (IMGs) and the Types of IMGs." In *International Medical Graduates in the United States: A Complete Guide to Challenges and Solutions,* edited by Hassaan Tohid and Howard Maibach, 1–12. Switzerland: Springer Press.

Gutiérrez, Elena R. 2008. *Fertility Matters: The Politics of Mexican Origin Women's Reproduction.* Austin: University of Texas Press.

Hall, Roberta M., and Bernice R. Sandler. 1982. "The Classroom Climate: A Chilly One for Women?" Washington, DC: Association of American Colleges.

Hannon, Lance, and Robert DeFina. 2016. "Reliability Concerns in Measuring Respondent Skin Tone by Interviewer Observation." *Public Opinion Quarterly* 80(2): 534–41.

Hargrove, Taylor, and Shannon Malone Gonzalez. 2022. "A Conversation on Race and Colorism in Social Forces." *Social Forces* 101(1): 102–10.

Hayes-Bautista, David E., and Roberto Chiprut. 2008. *The Art of Healing Latinos: Firsthand Accounts from Physicians and Other Health Advocates.* 2nd ed. Los Angeles: UCLA Chicano Studies Research Center Press.

Hoffman, Kelly M., Sophie Trawalter, Jordan R. Axt, and M. Norman Oliver. 2016. "Racial Bias in Pain Assessment and Treatment Recommendations, and False Beliefs about Biological Differences between Blacks And Whites." *Proceedings of the National Academy of Sciences* 113(16): 4296–4301.

Holmes, Seth M. 2013. *Fresh Fruit, Broken Bodies: Migrant Farmworkers in the United States.* Berkeley: University of California Press.

———. 2012. "The Clinical Gaze in the Practice of Migrant Health: Mexican Migrants in the United States." *Social Science and Medicine* 74(6): 873–81.

Holvino, Evangelina. 2010. "Intersections: The Simultaneity of Race, Gender and Class in Organizations Studies." *Gender, Work & Organization* 17(3): 277–84.

Hondagneu-Sotelo, Pierrette. 1992. "Overcoming Patriarchal Constraints: The Reconstruction of Gender Relations among Mexican Immigrant Women and Men." *Gender and Society* 6(3): 393–415.

———. 1994. *Gendered Transitions: Mexican Experiences of Immigration.* Berkeley: University of California Press.

Hsin, Amy, and Yu Xie. 2014. "Explaining Asian Americans' Academic Advantage Over Whites." *Proceedings of the National Academy of Sciences* 111(23): 8416–21.

Hulko, Wendy. 2009. "The Time and Context Contingent Nature of Intersectionality and Interlocking Oppressions." *Affilia: Journal of Women and Social Work* 24(1): 44–55.

Hunt, Linda M. 2005. "Beyond Cultural Competence: Applying Humility to Clinical Settings." In *The Social Medicine Reader*, edited by Gail E. Henderson et al., 133–35. Durham: Duke University Press.

Hurtado, Aida. 2006. "Un Cuadro—A Framing." In *Flor y Ciencia: Chicanas in Science, Mathematics and Engineering*, edited by Norma E. Cantu, 1–10. Washington, DC: The Adelante Project, AAAS.

Hyun, Jane. 2005. *Breaking the Bamboo Ceiling: Career Strategies for Asians.* New York: Harper Collins Publishers.

Irigoyen, Matilde, and Ruth E. Zambrana. 1979. "Foreign Medical Graduates (FMGs): Determining Their Role in the U.S. Health Care System." *Social Science and Medicine* 13A: 773–83.

Jolly, Paul. 2005. "Medical School Tuition and Young Physicians' Indebtedness." *Health Affairs* 24: 527–35.

Jenks, Angela C. 2011. "From 'Lists of Traits' to 'Open-Mindedness': Emerging Issues in Cultural Competence Education." *Culture, Medicine and Psychiatry* 35(2): 209–35.

Jenkins, Tanya. 2021. *Doctors' Orders: The Making of Status Hierarchies in an Elite Profession*. New York: Columbia University Press.

Johnson, Dawn R. 2012. "Campus Racial Climate Perceptions and Overall Sense of Belonging Among Racially Diverse Women in STEM Majors." *Journal of College Student Development* 53(2): 336–46.

Julliard, Kell, Josefina Vivar, Carlos Delgado, Eugenio Cruz, Jennifer Kabak, and Heidi Sabers. 2008. "What Latina Patients Don't Tell Their Doctors: A Qualitative Study." *Annals of Family Medicine* 6(6): 543–49.

Kaplan, Mitchell A., and Antonio Zavaleta. 2017. "Cultural Competency The Key to Latino Health Policy: A Commentary." *Journal of Hispanic Policy*. https://hjhp.hkspublications.org/2017/03/23/cultural-competency-the-key-to-latino-health-policy-a-commentary.

Kibria, Nazli. 1993. *Family Tightrope: The Changing Lives of Vietnamese Americans*. Princeton: Princeton University Press.

Kim, Yeonwoo, and Esther J. Calzada. 2019. "Skin Color and Academic Achievement in Young, Latino Children: Impacts across Gender and Ethnic Group." *Cultural Diversity and Ethnic Minority Psychology* 25(2): 220–31.

Krosgstad, Manuel Jens, and Ana Gonzalez-Barrera. 2015. "A Majority of English-Speaking Hispanics in the U.S. Are Bilingual." Washington, DC: Pew Research Center.

Kochnar, Rakesh, and Anthony Cilluffo. 2018. "Income Inequality Rising in the U.S. Is Rising Most Rapidly Among Asians." Washington, DC: Pew Research Center.

Kwon, Eugena, and Tracey L. Adams. 2018. "Choosing a Specialty: Intersections of Gender and Race among Asian and White Women Medical Students in Ontario." *Canadian Ethnic Studies Journal* 50(3): 49–68.

Kwon, Hyeyoung. 2015. "Intersectionality in Interaction: Immigrant Youth Doing American from an Outsider-Within Position." *Social Problems* 62(4): 623–41.

Laundry Workers Center. 2018. "Report on Working Conditions in the Retail Laundromat Industry." https://laundryworkerscenter.org/wp-content/uploads/2018/06/Eng-Laundry-Workers-Center-Report-2.pdf.

Lee, Jennifer, and Min Zhou. 2015. *The Asian American Achievement Paradox*. New York: Russell Sage Foundation.

Lee, Jennifer C., and Sarah J. Hatteberg. 2015. "Bilingualism and Status Attainment among Latinos." *Sociological Quarterly* 56(4): 695–722.

Lee, Jennifer J., and Janice M. McCabe. 2021. "Who Speaks and Who Listens: Revisiting the Chilly Climate in College Classrooms." *Gender and Society* 35(1): 32–60.

Loizate Achotegui, Joseba. 2009. "Estrés Limite y Salud Mental: El Síndrome del Inmigrante con Estres Crónico y Múltiple (Sindrome de Ulises)." *Gaceta Medica de Bilbao* 106(4): 122–33.

Lombarts, Kiki M. J., and Abraham Verghese. 2022. "Medicine is Not Gender-Neutral—She Is Male." *The New England Journal of Medicine* 385(13): 1284–87.

López, Andrea, Kristin S. Hoeft, Claudia Guerra, Judith C. Barker, Lisa H. Chung, and Nancy J. Burke. 2022. "Spanish-Speaking Mexican-American Parents' Experiences While Navigating the Dental Care System for Their Children." *Journal of Public Health Dentistry* 82: 99–104.

López, Nancy. 2002. *Hopeful Girls, Troubled Boys: Race and Gender Disparity in Urban Education*. New York: Routledge.

———. 2005. "Homegrown: How the Family Does Gender." In *Gender Through the Prism of Difference,* edited by Maxine Baca Zinn, Pierrette Hondagneu-Sotelo, and Michael A. Messner, 465–80. Oxford: Oxford University Press.

Lopez, Susan. 2020. "Black and Brown Doctors (Like Me) Are Not OK Right Now." *HuffPost*. https://www.huffpost.com/entry/black-brown-doctors-during-covid-19-pandemic_n_5fd125fac5b68ce17184d228.

Lorber, Judith. 1984. *Women Physicians: Career, Status, and Power*. London: Tavistock.

Lugo-Lugo, Carmen R. 2008. "'So You are a Mestiza?': Exploring the Consequences of Ethnic and Racial Clumping in the US Academy." *Ethnic and Racial Studies* 31(3): 611–28.

Lu, Jackson G., Richard E. Nisbett, and Michael W. Morris. 2020. "Why East Asians But Not South Asians are Underrepresented in Leadership Positions in the United States." *Proceedings of the National Academy of Sciences* 117(9): 4590–4600.

Levinson, Wendy, and Nicole Lurie. 2004. "When Most Doctors Are Women: What Lies Ahead? *Annals of Internal Medicine* 141: 471–74.

Ly, Dan P. 2022. "Historical Trends in the Representativeness and Incomes of Black Physicians, 1900–2018." *Journal of General Internal Medicine* 37(5): 1310–12.

Magaña, Dalia. 2021. *Building Confianza: Empowering Latinas/os Through Transcultural Health Care Communication.* Columbus: Ohio State University Press.

Maghbouleh, Neda. 2017. *The Limits of Whiteness: Iranian American and the Everyday Politics of Race.* Palo Alto, CA: Stanford University Press.

Mallet, Marie, and Joanna Pinto-Coelho. 2018. "Investigating Intra-Ethnic Divisions among Latino Immigrants in Miami, Florida." *Latino Studies* 16(1): 1–22.

Martinez, Laura E., Gabriela Solis, Vianney Gomez, Julio Mendez-Vargas, Sonja F. M. Diaz, and David E Hayes-Bautista. 2019. "The Current State of the Latino Physician Workforce: California Faces a Severe Shortfall in Latino Resident Physicians." Los Angeles, CA: Latino Policy & Politics Initiative.

McCall, Leslie. 2005. "The Complexity of Intersectionality." *Signs: Journal of Women in Culture and Society* 30(3): 1771–1800.

Medina, Carlos, and Christian Manuel Posso. 2009. "Colombian and South American Immigrants in the United States of America: Education Levels, Job Qualifications and the Decision to Go Back Home." *Borradores de Economía* 572: 1–42.

Mendoza, Hadrian, Akihiko Masuda, and Kevin Swartout. 2015. "Mental Health Stigma and Self-Concealment as Predictors of Help-Seeking Attitudes among Latina/o College Students in the United States." *International Journal for the Advancement of Counselling* 37(3): 207–22.

Ménjivar, Cecilia. 2000. *Fragmented Ties: Salvadoran Immigrant Networks in America.* Berkeley: University of California Press.

Ménjivar, Cecilia, and Leisy J. Abrego. 2012. "Legal Violence: Immigration Law and the Lives of Central American Immigrants." *American Journal of Sociology* 117(5): 1380–1421.

Metzl, Jonathan M., and Helena Hansen. 2014. "Structural Competency: Theorizing a New Medical Engagement with Stigma and Inequality." *Social Science & Medicine* 103: 126–33.

Meyer, Jean-Baptiste, Jorge Charum, Dora Bernal, Jacques Gaillard, Jose Granés, John Leon, Alvaro Montenegro, Alvaro Morales, Carlos Murcia, and Nora Narvaez-Berthelemot. 1997. "Turning Brain Drain into Brain Gain: The Colombian Experience of the Diaspora Option." *Science, Technology and Society* 2(2): 285–315.

Misra, Joya, Ethel Mickey, Ember S. Kanelee, and Laurel Smith-Doerr. 2024. "Creating Inclusive Department Climates in STEM Fields: Multiple Faculty Perspectives on the Same Departments. *Journal of Diversity in Higher Education* 17(2): 176–89.

Molina, Melaine F., Adaira I. Landry, Anita N. Chary, and Sherri-Ann M. Burnett-Bowie. 2020. "Addressing the Elephant in the Room: Microaggressions in Medicine." *Annals of Emergency Medicine* 76(4): 387–91.

Molina, Natalia. 2006. *Fit to Be Citizens?: Public Health and Race in Los Angeles, 1879–1939*. Berkeley: University of California Press.

———. 2011. "Borders, Laborers, and Racialized Medicalization: Mexican Immigration and US Public Health Practices in the 20th Century." *American Journal of Public Health* 101(6): 1024–31.

Monk, Ellis P. 2021. "The Unceasing Significance of Colorism: Skin Tone Stratification in the United States." *Daedelus* 150(2): 76–90.

Murguia, Edward, and Edward E. Telles. 1996. "Phenotype and Schooling among Mexican Americans." *Sociology of Education* 69(4): 276–89.

Murti, Lata. 2012. "Who Benefits from the White Coat? Gender Differences in Occupational Citizenship among Asian-Indian doctors." *Ethnic and Racial Studies* 35(12): 2035–53.

———. 2014. "With and Without the White Coat: The Racialization of Southern California's Indian Physicians." PhD dissertation, University of Southern California.

Murtha, Jules, and Barbara Bekiesz. 2022. "Teaching Critical Race Theory in Medical School Could Improve Patient Outcomes." *MDLinx*. https://www.mdlinx.com/article/teaching-critical-race-theory-in-medical-school-could-improve-patient-outcomes/3Qhz86bfcN5BmQFNClkIDv.

Mukkamala, Shruti, and Karen L. Suyemoto. 2018. "Racialized Sexism/Sexualized Racism: A Multimethod Study of Intersectional Experiences of Discrimination for Asian American Women." *Asian American Journal of Psychology* 9(1): 32–46.

Noe-Bustamante, Luis, Ana Gonzalez-Barrera, Khadija Edwards, Lauren Mora, and Mark Hugo Lopez. 2021. "Majority of Latinos Say Skin Color

Impacts Opportunity in America and Shapes Daily Life." Washington, DC: Pew Research Center.

Oboler, Suzanne. 1995. *Ethnic Labels, Latino Lives: Identity and the Politics of (Re) Presentation in the United States*. Minnesota: University of Minnesota Press.

Ochoa, Gilda. 2004. *Becoming Neighbors in a Mexican American Community: Power, Conflict, and Solidarity*. Texas: University of Texas Press.

———. 2013. *Academic Profiling: Latinos, Asian Americans and the Achievement Gap*. Minneapolis: University of Minnesota Press.

Olivares-Urueta, Mayra. 2012. "The Latino/a Health Professions Pipeline: An Overview." *Hispanic Association of Colleges and Universities*.

Olszewski, Aleksandra E. 2022. "Narrative, Compassion, and Counter Stories." *American Journal of Ethics* 24(3): 212–27.

Ong, Maria. 2005. "Body Projects of Young Women of Color in Physics: Intersections of Gender, Race, and Science." *Social Problems* 52(4): 593–617.

Orellana, Marjorie. 2009. *Translating Childhoods: Immigrant Youth, Language and Culture*. New Brunswick, NJ: Rutgers University Press.

Ostfeld, Mara C., and Nicole D. Yadon. 2021. "Mejorando La Raza? The Political Undertones of Latinos' Skin Color in the United States." *Social Forces* 100(4): 1806–32.

Osuna, Steven. 2015. "Intra-Latina/Latino Encounters: Salvadoran and Mexican Struggles and Salvadoran–Mexican Subjectivities in Los Angeles." *Ethnicities* 15(2): 234–54.

Ovink, Sarah M. 2013. "'They Always Call me an Investment': Gendered Familism and Latina/o College Pathways." *Gender and Society* 28(2): 265–88.

Padilla, Amado. 1994. "Ethnic Minority Scholars, Research, and Mentoring: Current and Future Issues." *Educational Researcher* 23(4): 24–27.

Padilla, Felix. 1985. *Latino Ethnic Consciousness: The Case of Mexican Americans and Puerto Ricans in Chicago*. Notre Dame, IN: University of Notre Dame Press.

Parra, Michelle G., and Lorena Garcia. 2023. "I Have Tasted Freedom": An Intersectional Analysis of College-Going Latinas' Desire for and Meanings of Mobility." *Gender & Society* 37(2): 268–91.

Pérez, Jose O., and André L. Reis de Silva. 2019. "Cuban Medical Internationalism through a Feminist Perspective." *Contexto Internacional* 41(1): 65–88.

Pérez, Raúl. 2022. *The Souls of White Jokes: How Racist Humor Fuels White Supremacy*. Palo Alto, CA: Stanford University Press.

Pesquera, Beatriz M. 1993. "In the Beginning He Wouldn't Lift Even a Spoon: The Division of Household Labor." In *Building with Our Hands: New Directions in Chicana Studies*, edited by Adela de la Torre and Beatriz M. Pesquera, 181–95. Berkeley: University of California Press.

Picca, Leslie, and Joe Feagin. 2007. *Two-Faced Racism: Whites in the Backstage and Frontstage*. London: Routledge.

Pierce, Jennifer L. 1995a. *Gender Trials: Emotional Lives in Contemporary Law Firms*. Berkeley: University of California Press.

———. 1995b. "Rambo Litigators: Emotional Labor in a Male Dominated Job." In *Gender Trials: Emotional Lives in Contemporary Law Firms,* edited by Jennifer L. Pierce, 50–82. Berkeley: University of California Press.

Pirtle, Whitney Laster N. 2020. "Racial Capitalism: A Fundamental Cause of Novel Coronavirus (COVID-19) Pandemic Inequities in the United States." *Society for Public Health Education* 47(4): 504–08.

Portes, Alejandro, and Patricia Fernández-Kelly. 2008. "No Margin for Error: Educational and Occupational Achievement Among Disadvantaged Children of Immigrants." *The Annals of the American Academy of Political and Social Science* 620(1): 12–36.

Portillo, Shannon. 2010. "How Race, Sex, and Age Frame the Use of Authority by Local Government Officials." *Law and Social Inquiry* 35(3): 603–23.

Powell, Farran, and Ilana Kowarski. 2020. "10 Costs to Expect When Applying to Medical School." Accessed December 15, 2023. https://www.usnews.com /education/best-graduate-schools/top-medical-schools/slideshows/10-costs-to-expect-when-applying-to-medical-school?onepage.

Raffaelli, Marcela, and Stephanie Green. 2003. "Parent-Adolescent Communication About Sex: Retrospective Reports by Latino College Students." *Journal of Marriage and Family* 65(2): 474–81.

Rafferty, J., A. Tsikoudas, and B. C. Davis. 2007. "Ear Candling: Should General Practitioners Recommend It?" *Canadian Family Physician* 53(12): 2121–22.

Raudenbush, Danielle. 2021. "'We go to Tijuana to Double Check Everything': The Contemporaneous Use of Health Services in the U.S. and Mexico by Mexican Immigrants in the Border Region." *Social Science & Medicine* 270. https://doi.org/10.1016/j.socscimed.2020.113584.

Ray, Victor. 2019. "A Theory of Racialized Organizations." *American Sociological Review* 84(1): 26–53.

Rendón, Laura I., Amaury Nora, Ripsime Bledsoe, and Vijay Kanagala. 2019. *"Científicos* Latinxs: The Untold Story of Underserved Student Success in STEM Fields of Study." Center for Research and Policy in Education, The University of Texas at San Antonio.

Rendon, Maria. 2019. *Stagnant Dreamers: How the Inner City Shapes the Integration of Second-Generation Latinos.* New York: Russell Sage Foundation.

Reskin, Barbara, and Patricia A. Roos. 1990. *Job Queues, Gender Queues: Explaining Women's Inroads into Male Occupations.* Philadelphia: Temple University Press.

Ridgeway, Cecilia L. 2014. "Why Status Matters for Inequality." *American Sociological Review* 79(1): 1–16.

Rincón, Lina. 2015. "Between Nations and the World: Negotiating Legal and Social Citizenship in the Migration Process: The Case of Colombian and Puerto Rican Computer Engineers in the American Northeast." PhD dissertation, State University of New York at Albany.

———. 2017. "The Indelible Effects of Legal Liminality Among Colombian Migrant Professionals in the United States." *Latino Studies* 15(3): 323–40.

Rincón, Lina, Johana Londoño, Jennifer Harford Vargas, and Maria Elena Cepeda. 2020. "Reimagining US Colombianidades: Transnational Subjectivities, Cultural Expressions, and Political Contestations." *Latino Studies* 18(3): 301–25.

Rodarte, Patricia, Jorge Garavito, Giancarlo Medina Pérez, Michael Farias, and Victor H. Hernandez. 2023. "Strategies to Increase the Spanish-Speaking Workforce in Orthopaedic Surgery within the United States." *The Journal of Bone and Joint Surgery.* DOI: 10.2106/JBJS.23.00631.

Romano, Max J. 2018. "White Privilege in a White Coat: How Racism Shaped My Medical Education." *Annals of Family Medicine* 16(3): 261–63.

Rosales, Rocío. 2020. *Fruteros: Street Vending, Illegality and Community in Los Angeles.* Berkeley: University of California Press.

Rosas, Ana. 2014. *Abrazando El Espiritú.* Berkeley: University of California Press.

Roth, Wendy. 2016. "The Multiple Dimensions of Race." *Ethnic and Racial Studies* 39(8): 1310–38.

Sarawasti, Ayu. 2013. *Seeing Beauty, Sensing Race in Transnational Indonesia.* Honolulu: University of Hawai'i Press.

———. 2023. *Scarred: A Feminist Journey Through Pain*. New York: NYU Press.

Schut, Rebecca A. 2022. "Disaggregating Inequalities in the Career Outcomes of International Medical Graduates in the United States." *Sociology of Health & Illness* 44: 535–65.

———. 2023. "White Boys in White? Nativist Discrimination in the Medical Profession and the Reproduction of Intersectional Inequalities in High-Skill Occupations." Paper Presentation at the American Sociological Association, Philadelphia, PA.

Smiley, Richard A. Ruttinger, Clark Oliviera, Carrie M. Hudson, Laura R. Allgeyer, Richard Reneau, Kyrani A. Silvestre, Josephine H. Alexander, and Maryann Alexander. 2020. "The 2020 National Nursing Workforce Survey." *Journal of Nursing Regulation* 12(1): 1–96.

Smith, Robert C. 2005. *Mexican New York: Transnational Lives of New Immigrants*. Berkeley: University of California Press.

Solórzano, Daniel G., and Tara J. Yosso. 2002. "Critical Race Methodology: Counter-Storytelling as an Analytical Framework for Education Research." *Qualitative Inquiry* 8(1): 23–44.

Stanton-Salazar, Ricardo. 2011. "A Social Capital Framework for the Study of Institutional Agents and Their Role in the Empowerment of Low-Status Students and Youth." *Youth & Society* 43(3): 1066–1109.

Stanton-Salazar, Ricardo, and Sanford M. Dornbusch. 1995. "Social Capital and the Reproduction of Inequality: Information Networks among Mexican-Origin High School Students." *Sociology of Education* 68(2): 116–35.

Sue, Derald Wing. 2010. *Microaggressions in Everyday Life: Race, Gender, and Sexual Orientation*. Hoboken, NJ: John Wiley & Sons Inc.

Talamantes, Efrain, Karla Gonzalez, Carol M. Mangione, Gery Ryan, Alejandro Jimenez, Fabio Gonzalez, Seira Santizo Greenwood, David E Hayes-Bautista, and Gerardo Moreno. 2016. "Strengthening the Community College Pathway to Medical School: A Study of Latino Students in California." *Family Medicine* 48(9): 703–10.

Talamantes, Efrain, Mark C. Henderson, Tonya L. Fancher, and Fitzhugh Mullan. 2019. "Closing the Gap: Making Medical School Admissions More Equitable." *The New England Journal of Medicine*, 380(9): 803–5.

Taningco, Maria Teresa V. 2008. "Latinos in STEM Professions: Understanding Challenges and Opportunities for Next Steps. A Qualitative Study Using

Stakeholder Interviews." Los Angeles, CA: Tomas Rivera Policy Institute.

Teherani, Arianne, Karen Hauer, Alicia Fernandez, Talmadge E. King, and Catherine Lucey. 2018. "How Small Differences in Assessed Clinical Performance Amplify to Large Differences in Grades and Awards: A Cascade with Serious Consequences for Students Underrepresented in Medicine." *Academic Medicine* 93(9): 1286–92.

Telles, Edward E., and Vilma Ortiz. 2008. *Generations of Exclusion: Mexican Americans, Assimilation, and Race.* New York: Russell Sage Foundation.

Theobald, Brianna. 2019. *Reproduction on the Reservation: Pregnancy, Childbirth, and Colonialism in Long Twentieth Century.* Chapel Hill: The University of North Carolina Press.

Tiako, Max Jordan Nguemeni, Eugenia C. South, and Victor Ray. 2021. "Medical Schools as Racialized Organizations: A Primer." *Annals of Internal Medicine* 174(8): 1143–45.

Tiako, Max Jordan Nguemeni, Victor Ray, and Eugenia C. South. 2022. "Medical Schools as Racialized Organizations: How Race-Neutral Structures Sustain Racial Inequality in Medical Education—A Narrative Review." *Journal of General Internal Medicine* 37(9): 2259–66.

Torres, Ivy R., Sarah Shklanko, Cynthia Haq, and Alana M.W. LeBron. 2022. "Occupational Health Within the Bounds of Primary Care: Factors Shaping the Health of Latina/o Immigrant Workers in Federally Qualified Health Centers." *American Journal of Industrial Medicine* 65(6): 468–82.

Tsai, Jennifer, and Ann Crawford-Roberts. 2017. "A Call for Critical Race Theory in Medical Education." *Academic Medicine* 92(8): 1072–73.

Uzogara, Ekeoma E. 2019. "Gendered Racism Biases: Associations of Phenotypes with Discrimination and Internalized Oppression Among Latinx American Women and Men." *Race and Social Problems* 11: 80–92.

Valenzuela, Abel Jr. 1999. "Gender Roles and Settlement Activities Among Children and Their Immigrant Families." *American Behavioral Scientist* 42(4): 720–42.

Valian, Virginia. 1999. *Why So Slow? The Advancement of Women.* Cambridge, MA: MIT Press.

Valle, Ariana J. 2019. "Race and the Empire-state: Puerto Ricans' Unequal U.S. Citizenship." *Sociology of Race and Ethnicity* 5(1): 26–40.

Vallejo, Jody Agius. 2012. *Barrios to Burbs: The Making of the Mexican-American Middle Class.* Palo Alto, CA: Stanford University Press.

Vasquez, Jessica M. 2011. *Mexican Americans Across Generations: Immigrant Families, Racial Realities*. New York: New York University Press.

Vasquez-Tokos, Jessica, and Kathryn Norton-Smith. 2016. "Talking Back to Controlling Images: Latinos' Changing Responses to Racism over the Life Course." *Ethnic and Racial Studies* 40(6): 912–30.

Vega, William A., Michael A. Rodriguez, and Alfonso Ang. 2010. "Addressing Stigma of Depression in Latino Primary Care Patients." *General Hospital Psychiatry* 32(2): 182–91.

Vogt, Rainbow, and Maria Teresa Taningco. 2008. "Latina & Latino Nurses: Why are There So Few?" Los Angeles, CA: Tomas Rivera Policy Institute.

Waters, Mary C. 1996. "The Intersection of Gender, Race, and Ethnicity in Identity Development of Caribbean American Teens." In *Urban Girls: Resisting Stereotypes, Creating Identities,* edited by Bonnie J. R. Leadbeater and Niobe Way, 65–81. New York: New York University Press.

———. 2001. *Black Identities: West Indian Immigrant Dreams and American Realities*. Cambridge, MA: Harvard University Press.

Williams, Christine. 1992. "The Glass Escalator: Hidden Advantages for Men in the 'Female' Professions." *Social Problems* 39(3): 253–67.

Wingfield, Adia Harvey. 2012. *No More Invisible Man: Race and Gender in Men's Work*. Philadelphia, PA: Temple University Press.

———. 2019. *Flatlining: Race, Work, and Health Care in the New Economy*. Berkeley: University of California Press.

———. 2020. "When Passion Serves a Purpose: Race, Social Networks and Countering Occupational Discrimination." In *The Ecology of Purposeful Living Across the Lifespan,* edited by Anthony L. Burrow and Patrick L. Hill, 183–97. New York: Springer.

Wingfield, Adia Harvey, and Renee Skeete Alston. 2014. "Maintaining Hierarchies in Predominantly White Organizations: A Theory of Racial Tasks." *American Behavioral Scientist* 58(2): 274–87.

Wingfield, Adia H., and Koji Chavez. 2020. "Getting In, Getting Hired, Getting Sideways Looks: Organizational Hierarchy and Perceptions of Racial Discrimination." *American Sociological Review* 85(1): 31–57.

Wolf, Diane L. 1997. "Family Secrets: Transnational Struggles Among Children of Filipino Immigrants." *Sociological Perspectives* 40(3): 457–82.

World Health Organization Global Health Workforce Statistics. 2023. "Physicians (per 1,000 people)—United States." Accessed October 16, 2023. https://data.worldbank.org/indicator/SH.MED.PHYS.ZS?locations=US.

Xierali, Imam M., and Marc A. Nivet. 2018. "The Racial and Ethnic Composition and Distribution of Primary Care Physicians." *Journal of Health Care for the Poor and Underserved* 29(1): 556–70.

Youngclaus, James, and Julie A. Fresne. 2020. "Physician Education Debt and the Cost to Attend Medical School." Washington, DC: Association of American Medical Colleges.

Zambrana, Ruth Enid, and Sylvia Hurtado. 2015. *The Magic Key: The Educational Journey of Mexican Americans from K-12 to College and Beyond.* Austin: University of Texas Press.

Zamora, Sylvia. 2022. *Racial Baggage: Mexican Immigrants and Race Across the Border.* Palo Alto, CA: Stanford University Press.

Zelek, Barbara, and Susan P. Phillips. 2003. "Gender and Power: Nurses and Doctors in Canada." *International Journal for Equity in Health* 2(1): https://doi.org/10.1186/1475-9276-2-1.

Zewude, Rahel, and Malika Sharma. 2021. "Critical Race Theory in Medicine." *Canadian Medical Association Journal* 193(20): E739–41.

Zhou, Min, and Carl L. Bankston. 1998. *Growing up American: How Vietnamese Children Adapt to Life in the United States.* New York: Russell Sage Foundation.

Zhou, M., and S. S. Kim. 2006. "Community Forces, Social Capital, and Educational Achievement: The Case of Supplementary Education in the Chinese and Korean Immigrant Communities." *Harvard Educational Review* 76(1): 1–29.

Zinn, Maxine Baca. 1979. "Political Familism: Toward Sex Role Equality in Chicano Families." *Aztlán: A Journal of Chicano Studies* 6(1): 13–26.

———. 2001. "Insider Field Research in Minority Communities." In *Contemporary Field Research,* edited by Robert M. Emerson, 159–166. Long Grove: Waveland Press.

Zinn, Maxine Baca, and Ruth Enid Zambrana. 2019. "Chicanas/Latinas Advance Intersectional Thought and Practice." *Gender & Society* 33(5): 677–701.

# Index

Asian-Canadian women medical professionals, 18, 248n15

Asians, 235n25; doctors, perceptions about, 166; Indian women, 44; median parental income of students, 242n23; medical graduates, 69; registered nurses, 247n12; women, 167

aspirations, 109

Association of American Medical Colleges (AAMC), 12

authority and age, 142–46

autonomy and independence for Latino/as, 43–44

backstage racism against light-skinned doctors, 162–64

Baez, Carolina, Dr., 238–39n7

Bankston, Carl L., 240n31

Bañuelos, Maricela, 245n6

Bashi, Vilna, 94, 245n5

Beagan, Brenda, 234–35n14

Becker, Howard, 6, 89

Bekiesz, Barbara, 252n2

Bhatt, Wasudha, 19

bias, 99, 135, 194; cultural, 97, 98, 222; gender, 43, 55, 80, 143; and phenotype, 16; racial, 65–66, 68, 116, 168, 180; racially, 14; in speciality selection, 112–18; status, 9, 137, 148, 149–50, 211

bilingualism: and colorism, 173–74; and culturally competent care during COVID-19 pandemic, 224–26; and gender, 4–5, 234n13; higher compensation for, 220; Latina doctors and cultural taxation, 126–32, 162; as linguistic capital, 107–9. *see also*

communication; language; linguistic capital

*The Birth of the Clinic* (Foucault), 235n20

black bag, 235n19

Blacks: male nurses, 170; medical students, 69, 70–71, 242n23; patients, 198, 252n2; physicians, 11, 19–20, 127, 152, 165, 236n30; registered nurses, 247n12

Black/white binary schema, 176

Bourdieu, Pierre, 102

*Boys in White* (Becker, Geer, Hughes, and Strauss), 6, 83, 191

Bracero Program (1942-1964), 7, 85

Brewer, Alexandra, 235n21

bridging capital, 102

Browne, Irene, 213

brown mestizas, 171

brown mestizos, 172, 173

bullying, 172

Burnett-Bowie, Sherri-Ann M., 247n13

burnout, 205, 226

Calderon, Enrique, Dr., 213

California College Promise Grant, 240n27

California community college, 240n27

California Medical Assistance Program, 255n50

California Promise Scholarship, 50

2001 California provision, 71

Canada, physicians in, 234–35n14

capitalistic ambitions, 46–47

Caraves, Yadira, Dr., 209

career choices, 5–6. *see also* gendered career choices

Caribbean migrants: cultural conceptions of identity, 252n50; women physicians, 239n9

Cassell, Joan, 10, 116, 134, 147

Central and South American women, gendered career-oriented messages from, 39–42

Certification Commission for Healthcare Interpreters (CCHI), 243n40

Chary, Anita N., 247n13

Chávez, Koji, 19–20

Chávez, Maria, 32, 43

Chinese doctors, 166

Chiprut, Roberto, 254n34

circuitous pathways: additional testing, costs, and requirements, 64, 66–70; barriers leading to, 60–62, 64; having a doctor parent, 82–83, 87; introduction, 59–60; majoring in non-STEM fields, 77–79; not having a doctor parent, 70–75; positively selected Latin American IMGs, 84–90; pre-health requirements, 80–82; weeder courses, 75–77

Cisneros, Sandra, 31

citizenship status, 176

Civil Rights Movement, 13

class privilege, 66, 158–59, 172

code-switching, 21

co-ethnic colleagues, 117, 119–20

co-ethnic gatekeepers, 97–98

co-ethnic male doctors, 124

co-ethnic mentorship, 102–3, 106

collective experience in medical school, 76–77

college-going behaviors of Latino/as, 44

Collins, Patricia Hill, 251n43

colorism: backstage racism encountered by light-skinned doctores, 162–64; immigrant shadow, 169–73; and language, 173–78; within Latinidad, 15–16; privileged marginality, 155–62; racialization in science, 164–68; varying skin tones and discrimination, 153–55; vignette, 151–53

communication, 156; and language incompetence, 128; between physician and patient, 146, 192, 254n37. see also bilingualism

community clinics, quality of care in. see physicians and patients of color, structural competency approach

community colleges, 50, 80–81, 103, 113, 240n27

community forums, 223–24

competence and age, 142–46

competitiveness in STEM classes, 76–77

Conrad 30 waiver program, 15, 237n49

continuity of care, 184, 186

Contreras, Lorenzo Servando, Dr., 2–3, 4

controlling images, 53, 160, 171, 251n43

cosmetic surgeries, 236n29

costs of medical education, 241n8, 242n15, 242n20; in Latin America, 86–87; medical College Admission Test (MCAT) fee, 241n8, 242n15; in the US, 66–69; for USMLE, 243n43

COVID-19 pandemic: anti-Asian hate crimes during, 251n38; culturally competent care during, 221–26

coworkers: co-ethnic, 117, 119–20; co-ethnic male, 124; racial microaggressions by, 168–70

critical consciousness, 94, 96, 245n6

critical race theory (CRT), 26–27, 252n2

cross-border health-seeking behaviors, 185

cross-category interactions, 137

cross-cultural linguistic needs, 183–86

Cuba: doctor-to-patient ratio, 213–14; gender composition in medicine, 25; medicine in, 214–19

Cuban Adjustment Act of 1966, 217

Cultural and Linguistically Appropriate Services (CLAS), 186

cultural beliefs, 132, 190

cultural biases, 97, 98, 222

cultural brokers, children as, 191, 233n1

cultural capital, 70, 71, 73, 79, 83

cultural competency: in building trust, 132; in diabetes management, 197–98; and training in medical school, 189, 190–91, 206–8; and treatment of minority patients, 158, 194–96; and unpaid labor, 126–32. *see also* culturally competent care

cultural exploitation at the workplace, 127

cultural expressions, 191–92

cultural humility, 194

cultural knowledge, 115, 155

culturally biased tests, 97, 98

culturally competent care, 182, 183–89; during pandemic, 221–26. *see also* cultural competency

culturally congruent care, 30, 212

culturally deficient assumptions, 98, 196–97

cultural metaphors, 189, 192

cultural norms and sexuality, 53

cultural pedagogies, 191

cultural racism, 192–93, 194–95

cultural status beliefs, 135–39

cultural taxation of Latina physicians, 126–32

curious feminist, 4, 136, 210

curriculum, medical schools, 103, 104, 106, 111, 194–95, 207

DACA for undocumented students, 242n29

darker-skinned Latinas/os, 16, 144, 154, 157, 161, 176–77, 211

Defense of Marriage Act (DOMA), 245n11

deference acts, 125–26, 134

2012 Deferred Action for Childhood Arrivals program, 71

delays in schooling, 74

Delgado, Marisa, Dr., 221–23

demeanor acts, 125–26, 146–47

demographic questionnaire, 154

Department of Health and Human Services, 185–86

devaluation, 10

diabetes management, cultural competence in, 197–98

Diablo Community College, 103

diet, addressing, 197–98

disdain, 164

disrespect, 140, 142, 145, 153, 196, 247n13

doctor parents, 82–83, 87

Dohan, Daniel, 239n12

Dominican physicians, 69, 213

Don Bosco Technical School's Architecture and Construction Engineering technology program, 239n10

double jeopardy, 236n33

double majoring, 78

downward social mobility, 39, 84, 239n12, 243–44n46

*Dr. 90210* (reality series), 236n29

dual queuing process, 248n16

Duany, Jorge, 252n50

Duran, Rosa, Dr., 1–2, 4–5

East Asians: immigrants, 105; in medicine, 166

Educational Commission for Foreign Medical Graduates (ECFMG) certification, 236–37n47

educational debt, 68–69, 89

educational hierarchy, 96

El Instituto Cultural Oaxaca, 26, 191

elite training positions, 101

El Palacio de Justicia, Bogota, Colombia, 243n39

emergency medical education, 235n21

emotion management, 146–50

empowerment agents, 96, 102–3; panethnic-based programs as, 109, 111–12. *see also* institutional agents

English language proficiency, 72

Enloe, Cynthia, 234n5

Enriquez, Laura, 71

equity work, 126–27; gendered, 127–32

Estrada, Emir, 234n12

ethnic affiliation, 159–60

ethnic-affirming spaces, 98

ethnic hostility against South Asians, 251n38

ethnic identity, revelation of, 171–72

ethnic markers, 154

ethnic medical organizations, 111

ethnic-themed housing programs, 109

exclusion from coworkers, 129

experiential knowledge, 27, 94, 245n6

extended family members and career choices, 47–48

Fadiman, Anne, 190

familial financial providers, men as, 42–43

familial obligations, 10, 44, 238–39n7, 247n12

familism/*familismo*, 35, 55, 239n15

family dynamics, 240n31, 252–53n4

family medicine, 113

family members, accompanying to provider's office, 253n18

*Family Secrets* (González-López), 238n5

feedback, 115–16, 158

fees. *see* costs of medical education

female chaperones, 248n19, 255n45

femininity: and competence, 144; and identity, 125

feminist theories and racialized organizations, 17–20

Fernández, Raul, 237–38n69

Fernández-Kelly, Maria Patricia, 244n1

financial aid, 61

financial support: from family, 68–69, 83, 247n12; to family, 43, 44, 72, 75, 89

first-generation college students, 12, 90, 106, 108; bachelor's degrees for, 241n4; challenges of, 69–75; definition, 241n1; shadowing by, 246n23

*Foos in Medicine* (social media page), 245n4

forced sterilization of immigrant Latinas, 7, 251n43

Foucault, Michel, 235n20

Gálvez, Alysha, 196

Gándara, Patricia, 70

García, Gina, 247n42

García, Irvin, 245n4

García-López, Gladys, 140, 142–43

gatekeeping agents, encountering, 96–101

Geer, Blanche, 6

gender: biased double standard, 43; biases at work, 55, 130, 148; bias in education, 43, 80; and career choices, 4, 47–49, 116; discrimination in Latines, 240n26; gender-appropriate behavior, 134; gender-appropriate emotional labor, 146; hierarchy, 10, 136–37; imbalance in medical profession, 9–10; and interpretation work, 234n13; intersected with ethnicity, 108, 115–16; intersection with age, 142–44; order, discriminatory, 19, 134, 139; privilege, 32–33, 38, 133–34, 136, 138–39, 153, 157, 160, 177, 217; social mobility and time, 54–56; status beliefs, 135–39

gendered career choices: contradictory gendered ideologies, 33–39; gender, social mobility, and time, 54–56; gendered messages among Central and South American women, 39–42; introduction, 31–33; procuring financial and social independence from men, 42–49; sexual policing and monitoring, 49–53

gendered cultural expectations, 13, 240n31; and Central and South American women, 39–42; and socioeconomic position, 35

gendered cultural taxation, 126–32

gendered cultural tightropes, 35, 41, 55–56

gendered deference, 139; age, authority, and competence questioned, 142–46; cultural understandings of, 220; and demeanor in organizations, understanding, 124–26; emotion management, 146–50; gendered cultural taxation, 126–32; microaggressions from women nurses and staff, 133–42; vignette, 122–24

gendered division of labor, 39–40, 252–53n4

gendered dynamics within Latine families, 31–33

gendered familism, 43

gendered identities, 16, 107, 125

gendered ideologies: contradictory, 33–39; evolving, 54–55; of familial incest, 238n5

gendered microaggressions, 124, 133–42, 149. see also microaggressions

gendered networks, 107–9

gendered networks and linguistic capital: benefits of, 94–95; encountering gatekeeping agents, 96–101; gendered networks, 107–9; men and social networks, 103–6; panethnic-based programs as empowerment agents, 109, 111–12; really significant others, 102–3; specialty selection, 112–21; STEM faculty mentors, dearth of, 95–96; vignette, 92–94

gendered processes, 213–14

gendered racism, 126, 146–48; from support staff, 138–39

gender inequality, 9, 34, 235n21; and cultural competence, 126–32

gender-related stressors, 13

Immigrant Syndrome with Chronic and Multiple Stress, 198

Immigration Reform and Control Act (1986), 72

Indian doctors, 19, 70–71, 104, 166. *see also* Asians; South Asians

inequality, 18, 176

institutional agents, 96, 97, 102–3, 115. *see also* empowerment agents

institutionalized discrimination, 89, 95

institutional support, 96

Interested Governmental Agency, 15

interlocutors, children as, 1–2

internalized racism, 16, 53

international medical graduates (IMGs): advantages over Americans, 65–66; advantages over Latina/o USMGs, 60, 84–90, 210–11, 216–17; extended exchange visitor (J) visas to, 237n48–49; and gatekeepers, 100; Latin American, 83, 210, 213; Latin American, positively selected, 84–90; questioning of competence of, 173; United States Medical Licensing Exam (USMLE) for, 69, 236n45; US citizenship for, 236n46

interpersonal skills, 115–16, 132

interpreters/interpretation, 107; children as, 1–2, 191; cultural taxation of, 126–28; and gender, 126–28, 234n13; medical, 6–7, 186, 187, 243n40; Mexican-origin girls as, 234n12

intersectionality/intersections, 8–9, 12, 17, 19, 27, 28–30, 115–20, 134–35, 142, 145, 153, 172, 182, 210, 219, 236n33

intragroup distinctions, 14–17

intra-racial stratification, 176, 251n33

J 1 (extended exchange visitor) visas, 15, 84, 237n48–49, 243–44n46

jealousy, 144

Jenkins, Tanya M., 86, 100–101

Jones Act of 1917, 249n3

*Journal of the American Medical Association*, 10

Julliard, Kell, 255n45

K-9 schooling, 88, 216

K-12 education, 12, 61, 89, 244n1

Kwon, Eugena, 18, 248n15

Landry, Adaira I., 247n13

language: assistance competence, 186; broker, children as, 1–2, 4; codes, 254n32; and colorism, 173–78; cues, 191. *see also* bilingualism; linguistic capital

Latina/o: majoring in non-STEM fields, 77–79; parental pressures to be financially independent, 48–49; representation in medicine, 209–11, 213–14

Latina/o Critical Race Theory (LatCrit), 27

Latina/o physicians: about, 6–8; broader context of being, 11–13; clinical shadowing for interviews, 25–27; demographic statistics by sex, 228–29; ethnic capital resources of, 211; experiences during the pandemic, 221–26; financial assistance to family, 66; findings from interviews with, 20–22; gendered dynamics and inequality, 213–14; intra-Latine focus, 211–13; medicine in Cuba as a counterpoint, 214–19; physician

misapprehensions, 164

misguided information, 112

Misra, Joya, 127

Molina, Natalia, 7, 247n13

Monk, Ellis P., 15–16

moral harm, 207

multigenerational punishment, 71–72

Murtha, Jules, 252n2

Murti, Lata, 19, 129, 166

National Board of Certified Medical
   Interpreters (NBCMI), 243n40

National Hispanic Medical Association
   (NHMA), 11, 102

National Latino and Latina Physician
   Day, 209

National Medical Association (NMA),
   236n30

National Nursing Workforce Survey,
   134

National Service Corps Program, 113

Native American women, 235n18

nativist credentialism, 84, 243n44

navigational capital, 94

Nicaragua: immigrants, 71, 169, 222;
   Temporary Protected Status in,
   242n28

nurses: Asian-Canadian women medical
   professionals' interaction with,
   248n15; and Black physicians, 127;
   collaboration with physicians, 247n13;
   Hispanic, 133; interactions with
   physicians, 18–19, 248n15; lack of
   Spanish competence and patient
   interaction, 128; Latina, 131, 133–34, 135;
   as medical interpreters, 187; microaggressions toward Latina physicians,
   133–42, 149; registered, 134, 247n12;

verbal abuses from, 248n15; and white
   women surgeons, 10

nursing, Latinas/os opting for, 247n12


Oaxacan Triqui agricultural laborers,
   181–82

Obama, Barack, 71

observed race, 158

Ocasio, Soraida, Dr., 239n9

occupational citizenship, 19

occupational hierarchy, 12, 128

occupational label, 210

occupational sex segregation, 9–10

occupational status, 168

offsetting gender disadvantage, 46–49

Olszweski, Aleksandra, 182

Ong, Mia, 18

ophthalmologists, 246n35

oppressive gendered dynamics, 36

optometrists, 246n35

organizational hierarchies, 18; and
   discrimination, 20

Ortiz, Vilma, 54–55

Ostfeld, Mara C., 250n15

Ovink, Sarah, 43, 44, 239n15


Padilla, Amado, 127

panethnic-based programs as empowerment agents, 109, 111–12

pan-ethnic labels, 14, 210

pan-ethnic solidarity, 14

parents: doctor, 82–83, 87; education of,
   34, 35, 54, 155; expectations of, 35;
   gendered career-oriented messages
   from, 32–38; pressures to be financially independent from, 48–49; social
   capital of, 83; socioeconomic position
   of, 55–56

structural competency. *see* physicians and patients of color, structural competency approach

structural discrimination, 16

structural limitations in health care systems, 9, 190, 201–2

study groups, 75, 78

*Survival of the Knitted* (Bashi), 245n5

taboos, 132

Talamantes, Efrain, Dr., 80

teaching assistants, 75

Teherani, Arianne, 246n36

Telles, Eddie, 54–55

Temporary Protected Status, 71, 242n28

test proficiency, 72–73

Theobald, Brianna, 235n18

"token" context, 226

Torres, Calliope, Dr., 238n4

Torres, Ivy, 189

traditional health beliefs, 190, 212

Triqui migrant patients, 190

trust: in children, 51–52; from Latine patients, 175; patients', 180; in US-based doctors, 6

tuition fee. *see* costs of medical education

tutoring, 78

Twine, France Winddance, 132

UC Berkeley's Molecular Cell Biology program, 104

UC-Cuba Academic Initiative, 214

Ulysses Syndrome, 198

underrepresented in medicine (URM), 14

undocumented immigrants, 255n48

United States (US): doctor-to-patient ratio, 213–14; medical workforce, control of, 14–15; racial classification system, 155; racial hierarchies, 158–59; schools, 14

United States medical graduates (USMGs), 19, 25, 238n4. *see also* Latina/o USMGs

United States Medical Licensing Examination (USMLE), 69, 85, 87, 100, 236–37n47; fee for, 243n43

unpaid labor, gendered, 126–32

upward social mobility, 74, 103, 210

urban public schools, 72

Valenzuela, Abel, 234n12

Valian, Virginia, 141

Valle, Ariana, 249n3

Vallejo, Jody Agius, 172

Vasquez-Tokos, Jessica, 36, 48, 238–39n7

victim blaming, 192–93

Vietnamese American women, 52

Vietnamese daughters, gendered expectations, 240n31

vocational jobs/pink-collar work, 114–15

volunteer coordinators, 96–97

wage gap and gender discrimination, 24–25

weeder courses, 75–77

West Indian immigrants, 94

white: heteropatriarchy, 6; male medical students, 69, 191; male physicians, 10, 235n27; median parental income of, 242n23; physicians as gatekeeping agents, 97; racial category, 177; racial privilege, 217, 235n27; supremacist ideologies, 162; upper-middle-class, 105

white-coat ceremonies, 235n20

white-dominated spaces, 170

whiteness of the occupation, 153

white-passing Latino physicians, 173

White People 4 Black Lives Matter (WP4BL), 160

white-presenting Latinas, 154, 173; physicians, 160–62

white-presenting Latino physicians, 155–62, 177

white women, 132; entrance into male-dominated workplaces, 248n16; gender discrimination and sexism against, 18; LGBTQ, 132; in medical profession, 9–10, 247n4; in positions of power, 167

Wingfield, Adia Harvey, 19–20, 71, 127, 165

within-group resource heterogeneity, 160

*The Woman in the Surgeon's Body* (Cassell), 10

women: IMGs, 85–86; and linguistic capital, 107–9; patients, 130. *see also* Latina physicians; Latinas

women nurses, microaggressions from, 144; discriminatory practices of, 133–34; Latina physicians' self-presentation, 139–42; status beliefs, 135–39

Women of All Red Nations (WARN), 235n18

women of color physicians, interaction with nurses, 18–19

*Women Physicians: Careers, Status and Power* (Lorber), 10

working-class immigrant family, physicians from: backstage racism against, 162–64; bridging capital of, 102; with college-educated parents, 155; debt on, 68–69, 89; homogeneous peer networks for, 105; racist microaggressions toward, 162–63, 169, 172; and socioeconomic position of parents, 55–56; specialty selection for, 119–20; stereotyping, 164–65; white-presenting, 160–61

working-class Latino immigrant family: college-going behaviors of Latino/as from, 44; first-generation college students from, 60–61, 70, 82; gendered ideologies of, 33–39; language codes among, 254n32

workplace: experiences for physicians of color, 19; infections/injuries to immigrant patients, 187–89; interactions, 18

Yadon, Nicole D., 250n15

Zambrana, Ruth Enid, 36–37

Zhou, Min, 240n31

Founded in 1893,
UNIVERSITY OF CALIFORNIA PRESS
publishes bold, progressive books and journals
on topics in the arts, humanities, social sciences,
and natural sciences—with a focus on social
justice issues—that inspire thought and action
among readers worldwide.

The UC PRESS FOUNDATION
raises funds to uphold the press's vital role
as an independent, nonprofit publisher, and
receives philanthropic support from a wide
range of individuals and institutions—and from
committed readers like you. To learn more, visit
ucpress.edu/supportus.

www.ingramcontent.com/pod-product-compliance
Lightning Source LLC
LaVergne TN
LVHW091522230525
812061LV00002B/165